MW00576244

"This is a timely book, ▯ now using aromatherapy ▯ provide the nurse and nurse-midwife with valuable information to be able to advise women about the safety of aromatherapy in maternity care.

I had the pleasure of working with Pam in the UK whilst she was completing a Masters' degree in Complementary Therapies at the University of Westminster, and I know that her focus is on safe and appropriate application of aromatherapy for pregnant and birthing women, supported by research evidence."

—*Denise Tiran, FRCM, MSc, RM, PGCEA,*
*Education Director at Expectancy*

"This book represents years of nursing and midwifery practice, research and education in women's health aromatherapy. The mainstream popularity of aromatherapy necessitates an expert nursing aromatherapy guide for the safest, most effective care of women pregnancy-postpartum.

I highly recommend this book as a resource to nurses and all women considering aromatherapy during the pregnancy-postpartum stages."

—*Birdie Gunyon Meyer, RN, MA Coordinator,*
*Perinatal Mood Disorders Program, Indiana University Health,*
*Past President of Postpartum Support International PSI*

"Pam Conrad gracefully combines both the art and science of aromatherapy. She has a profound knowledge about the clinical use of essential oils but also the artful use of aromatherapy in daily life.

As essential oils are so easily accessible as home remedies, it is very tempting to believe that there are no risks in using them. One main thing that I love and respect about Pam's teachings is that she puts safety first, especially for vulnerable patients like pregnant women, infants and young children.

As parents and patients use essential oils for conditions ranging from benign viral illnesses to advanced malignancies, it is paramount for any medical health practitioner to have at least basic knowledge of the benefits and safety of essential oils. I highly recommend Pam's book to all my colleagues and patients."

—Dr Alina Olteanu, MD, PhD, FAAP, ABIHM, Whole Child Texas

"Pam Conrad is a Purdue-trained nurse and valued NAHA Certified Clinical Aromatherapist®. In addition to being a registered nurse for over 25 years, Pam has studied abroad with aromatherapy icons like Jane Buckle, Denise Tiran, and Ethel Burns. Pam is passionate about supporting women's health and evidence-based aromatherapy. In 2008, Pam developed the first US evidence-based hospital Aromatic Childbirth® nursing curriculum.

There is a great need for practicing clinical nurses and therapists who follow an evidence-based approach combined with experience gained in clinical practice. It is wonderful to see NAHA members like Pam who are active in authoring books, participating in studies, and teaching."

—Annette Davis, ND, Certified Clinical Aromatherapist and Nutritionist,
President of National Association for Holistic Aromatherapy NAHA

"This is essential information to provide safe guidance for our families choosing to utilize aromatherapy. I use this valuable information on a daily basis."

—Stephanie VanderHorst, CNM, RN,
Past President of Indiana Association of Nurse Midwives

"Pam's course on aromatherapy for women's health has been so beneficial for me in my practice as a nurse. The education I received has allowed me to practice safe aromatherapy for my pregnant and laboring mommas!

Practicing clinically evidenced-based aromatherapy is a must in the hospital setting. By having a book to help guide this practice that can be referenced while at the bedside would be an invaluable asset to the aromatherapy world as it begins to be used more and more in hospitals alongside traditional medicine."

—Katlyn Devereux, RN, BSN, CMSRN, St. Elizabeth Medical Center

"Although there is an abundance of essential oil information flooding the market, very little is clinically evidenced-based and safe for perinatal use. In fact, much of the information is harmful. Pam Conrad's expertise and experience is what is needed for an OB/GYN aromatherapy guidebook for practicing professionals."

—*Kathy Ryan, RN, CCAP, Perinatal Support Services*
*St Vincent Women's Hospital*

"With the growing popularity of integrative medicine, essential oils have found their way back into health care. Historically anecdotal evidence or previous experience drove the choice of essential oils. However, it is not enough for an oil just to smell good; healthcare professionals must understand the oil's reported benefits, potential risks, and contraindications as well as the current state of associated research. This book provides the evidence-based foundation to practice evidence-based aromatherapy for medical professionals."

—*Dr Liz Nutter, CNM, DNP, RNC-OB*

*of related interest*

**Aromatherapy in Midwifery Practice**
*Denise Tiran*
ISBN 978 1 84819 288 1
eISBN 978 0 85701 235 7

**Complementary Therapies in Maternity Care:**
**An Evidence-Based Approach**
*Denise Tiran*
ISBN 978 1 84819 328 4
eISBN 978 0 85701 284 5

**Aromatherapy, Massage and Relaxation in Cancer Care**
**An Integrative Resource for Practitioners**
*Edited by Ann Carter and Dr Peter A. Mackereth*
ISBN 978 1 84819 281 2
eISBN 978 0 85701 228 9

# WOMEN'S HEALTH AROMATHERAPY

*A Clinically Evidence-Based Guide for Nurses, Midwives, Doulas and Therapists*

## PAM CONRAD
PGd, BSN, RN, CCAP

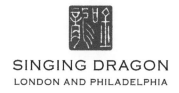

SINGING DRAGON
LONDON AND PHILADELPHIA

First published in 2019
by Singing Dragon
an imprint of Jessica Kingsley Publishers
73 Collier Street
London N1 9BE, UK
and
400 Market Street, Suite 400
Philadelphia, PA 19106, USA

*www.singingdragon.com*

**Library of Congress Cataloging in Publication Data**
Names: Conrad, Pam (Aromatherapist), author.
Title: Women's health aromatherapy : a clinically evidence-based guide for
    nurses, midwives, doulas, and therapists / Pam Conrad.
Description: London ; Philadelphia : Jessica Kingsley Publishers, 2019. |
    Includes bibliographical references.
Identifiers: LCCN 2018035843 | ISBN 9781848194250
Subjects: | MESH: Aromatherapy--methods | Women's Health | Evidence-Based
    Practice | Obstetrics | Gynecology
Classification: LCC RM666.A68 | NLM WA 309.1 | DDC 615.3/219-
-dc23 LC record available at https://lccn.loc.gov/2018035843

**British Library Cataloguing in Publication Data**
A CIP catalogue record for this book is available from the British Library

ISBN 978 1 84819 425 0
eISBN 978 0 85701 378 1

Printed and bound in Great Britain by Clays Ltd, Elcograf S.p.A.

Dedicated to *all women,* especially
my mother Shirley and daughter Katie

# Contents

# Contents

# Acknowledgements

Gratitude to all women, practitioners, girlfriends and patients who've walked with me on this 20-year aromatic journey and are the inspiration for this book. Special love to my daughter and mother for enduring countless aromatherapy preparations hidden in their purses and backpacks when all of their friends only used "normal" pharmaceutical remedies. Special thanks to my editor, James Cherry, who identified a gap for a clinically evidence-based aromatherapy guidebook for women's health practitioners and contacted me to share my years of nursing aromatherapy experience, and Victoria Peters and Maddy Budd for their editing guidance and expertise. Immense gratitude to all of the nurses, midwives, doulas and therapists who've been my students and to all of the women we've treated with aromatherapy who have shared their experiences with us. Heartfelt gratitude to the 28 brave women in our postpartum depression and anxiety aromatherapy research study whose results guide other women and practitioners with simple aromatherapy methods to help women suffering emotional distress in early motherhood.

Honored and grateful thanks to my mentors and teachers, Denise Tiran, Ethel Burns and Jane Buckle, international nursing and midwifery aromatherapy experts who initiated and enriched my journey in women's health nursing aromatherapy.

Special thanks go to my parents for a childhood in our family pharmacy focused on enhancing the health and well-being of others, and my brother, Dan, for showing me the importance of passion in your chosen path. And to my husband, Rod, whose love, friendship and constant support I truly cherish, and our children, Katie and Ryan, the treasures of my life, whose love, personal character and accomplishments inspire me and make me proud to be your mother!

# Key Terminology

| | |
|---|---|
| **Amenorrhea** | absence of monthly menstrual period (more common in runners, dancers and gymnasts and women with some eating disorders) |
| **Antepartum** | before birth |
| **Anticoagulant** | "blood thinning" medications affecting the clotting of blood |
| **Cardiac** | pertaining to the heart |
| **Carrier** | unscented lotion, oil or gel to dilute essential oils prior to skin application |
| **Cesarean section/ C-section** | childbirth by surgery |
| **Dysmenorrhea** | painful menstrual periods |
| **Eclampsia** | serious condition before, during or after delivery with symptoms of preeclampsia and onset of seizures: **high risk** |
| **Epidural** | anesthesia injected into the spinal epidural space for pain relief during labor |
| **Essential oil** | highly concentrated oils extracted and distilled from aromatic plants |
| **Established labor** | regular rhythmic contractions of the uterus and progressive dilation of the cervix |
| **Hemorrhage** | excess bleeding: **higher risk** |
| **Hot flashes** | rapid rise in heat sensation and increased perspiration associated with menopause/hormonal changes |
| **Infertility** | inability to conceive/become pregnant after one year of unprotected sexual intercourse |
| **Intrapartum** | during birth/labor and delivery |
| **Menarche** | very first menstrual cycle |

| | |
|---|---|
| **Menopause** | end of menstrual cycles (no period for one consecutive year); average age 51 |
| **Menorrhagia** | heavy menstrual periods |
| **Menses** | menstrual cycle/monthly period |
| **Miscarriage** | fetal/pregnancy loss prior to 20 weeks |
| **Night sweats** | heat sensations and perspiring at night associated with menopause/hormonal changes |
| **Perimenopause** | time prior to menopause as hormonal levels are shifting and menopausal symptoms are increasing (duration can be up to ten years) |
| **Pitocin/oxytocin induction** | IV medication to start/induce labor contractions: **no clary sage** |
| **Placenta previa** | placenta is positioned at the cervical opening prior to the fetus: **higher risk** |
| **Polyhydramnios** | excess amniotic fluid: **higher risk** |
| **Postpartum** | after giving birth |
| **Preeclampsia** | complication of pregnancy with elevated blood pressure, protein in urine, swelling/edema: **higher risk** |
| **Premenstrual syndrome/PMS** | various uncomfortable physical and emotional symptoms experienced by some women prior to the onset of menstrual period |
| **Prenatal/antenatal** | pregnancy prior to birth |
| **Preterm labor** | labor contractions prior to term: **higher risk** |
| **Pyrexia** | fever/elevated body temperature which may be a sign of infection |
| **Renal** | pertaining to kidneys |
| **Transverse, breech or unstable lie** | fetus not in head first position: **higher risk** |

# Introduction

A childhood spent in my father's pharmacy inspired my devotion to medicine and education, and a desire to help others achieve health and well-being with some type of remedy, pill or plant. Respecting the optimal amount of a proven medication to achieve the best outcome with the least amount of risk was just common sense. With strong ancestral roots, a path toward nursing was paved with intrigue and respect for all things medical, accompanied by a deep desire to experience and understand the human condition up close and personal.

After graduating from Purdue University in nursing, the road led to my first position at Texas Heart Institute and over the next three decades to roles as a trauma, psychiatric and women's health nurse. Absorbed with the drama of the human condition at its most vulnerable and the intrigue of medicine, I longed for the special knowledge and tools to fill the gaps of modern medicine. In the early days of holistic/preventive medicine, lifestyle practices were identified as probable risk factors for cardiac events and cancer. Inspired by these findings, I set out on a quest for educational opportunities in nutritional, herbal and stress-reducing modalities. An opportunity to study clinical aromatherapy for healthcare professionals was offered at Indiana University Medical Center and my education was enthusiastically supported by the IU Center of Excellence for Women's Health. A pleasant, clinically evidence-based modality for minor illnesses and injuries that eases common side effects of necessary medications and treatments while enhancing emotional well-being was a perfect fit.

In 2001 after I became a certified clinical aromatherapy practitioner (CCAP), we were transferred to England with my husband's job. I devoured all available books and clinical research on aromatherapy and women's health, which all had been authored by UK midwives and nurses. Once in England, I interned at Queen Mary's Hospital and prenatal clinic for one year with Denise Tiran, midwife, professor and international expert on aromatherapy in pregnancy and childbirth. With a focus to return to the US to practice and teach nurses bedside clinical aromatherapy, I acquired specialty knowledge and practical skills to provide complementary therapies to women to ease their discomforts and enhance their childbirth experiences. Additionally, I met and consulted with the Oxford midwives (Burns *et al.* 2000) who conducted an eight-year clinical study with 8058 women in labor who received aromatherapy treatments for pain, nausea, anxiety and contractions, and continue their program to this day. This experience and knowledge gained is the foundation for the Women's Health Clinical Aromatherapy course for nurses and midwives, the only clinically evidence-based course in the US for women's health nurses since 2008 and approved by the American Holistic Nurses Association, a division of the American Nurses Association. Hundreds of US nurses now safely practice clinically evidence-based aromatherapy with their patients in clinics and hospitals. The focus of this book is the results and lessons learned from 20 years of following the clinical aromatherapy evidence base in practice, developing curriculum for nurses and midwives, conducting research and sharing the data from more than 1500 aromatherapy treatments.

The world of aromatherapy has changed dramatically since I entered the field 20 years ago. A word of caution: the degree of current popularity of aromatherapy far exceeds the number of individuals formally educated in the field. There is a current trend toward strong multilevel essential oil company loyalty, daily consumption, overuse and exaggerated unsafe claims without adequate education and understanding. Women in pregnancy/

postpartum should avoid this type of aromatherapy. Nursing is the most trusted profession in our society through our competent caring, knowledge of current safe practice and patient advocacy. I'm writing this book after 20 years of nursing aromatherapy practice to share professionally what I know to be safe and effective with very minimal risk, and 30 years since the first study began on an obstetric (OB) unit in Oxford, England, there's not been a single serious incident involving any woman or infant. The clinical evidence base in this book provides the practitioner with proof and rationale for their essential oil and method options to ease patients' suffering. This is the standard of practice for nursing aromatherapy.

As a 30-year nurse and certified clinical aromatherapist for 20 years, I have treasured my ability to offer patients and educate nurses and midwives in the "caring comfort" tools of aromatherapy. The vast scope of women's emotional and physical health, often altered by hormonal imbalance, has always intrigued me as well as the multitude of positive responses I've witnessed with aromatherapy.

As a nurse, the frequently spoken "It's not yet time for your medication"—as an uncomfortable patient requested something for anxiety or pain—began a 20-year quest for complementary comfort measures for patient care. Clinical aromatherapy fills this gap in time and eases unnecessary suffering without potentiating risk factors or side effects.

Stressful lifestyles have been identified as the most common cause of progression of illness and increased risks of negative outcomes. Modern women, often in charge of personal and familial healthcare, are seeking alternative treatment and remedy choices for reasons of economics, trust, improved outcomes and reduced risks. In the past 20 years, multiple medical events have heightened awareness, decreased trust in the status quo and led to enhanced personal responsibility in healthcare choices. Hormonal, physical and psychological conditions and their standard treatments have all come under scrutiny. In 2002, the multicenter Women's Health Initiative (WHI) study ended prematurely as serious risk factors were identified with standard hormone replacement therapy (HRT) for menopause (Hersh, Stefanick and Stafford 2004). Manufacturers of common chronic pain medications have admitted that their previously unreleased data had shown increased cardiovascular risks with prolonged use of their medications (US Food and Drug Administration 2004). Select antidepressant medications appear to increase risks of suicide in young adults and are now required to have black-box warnings on their labels (Hammad 2006). Common side effects of routine pharmaceuticals are wreaking havoc on women's bodies. All of these recent events have decreased trust in traditional healthcare, led women to seek alternatives and enhanced the growth of complementary alternative medicine.

Aromatherapy is a complementary therapy related to herbal medicine, identified through archeological excavations from 60,000 years ago as the oldest known medicinal therapy for humans. Essential oils—"the tools of aromatherapy"—available on a small scale since the 1960s, have recently experienced an explosion of popularity with women seeking alternatives for the alleviation of stress, physical discomfort and hormonal upheaval. This book will differentiate the type of aromatherapy that uses products sold directly by lay individuals or in shops and that practiced by licensed healthcare professionals educated in clinical aromatherapy for the healthcare realm.

In the past decade, large competitive multilevel companies have sold millions of dollars' worth of essential oils to individuals with unsubstantiated claims of warding off illness and providing cures for a wide range of conditions without research studies or an evidence base to prove their claims. With aromatherapy gaining attention as a healing modality, it is now more readily available than in the past, which has many positive aspects. However, a belief in aromatherapy as a panacea for all conditions often overlooks potential risks of combining oils with modern pharmaceuticals and medical conditions. A bit of caution is advised for specific aromatherapy methods and oil selection with pregnancy, lactation, serious medical conditions and medications. Outlining the many benefits and specific risks with aromatherapy highlights the importance of the clinically evidence-based nursing and midwifery aromatherapy education that is found in this book.

Licensed healthcare professionals practice clinical aromatherapy as a specialty of nursing and midwifery with advanced education in aromatherapy for clinical conditions. Clinical aromatherapy is defined as the therapeutic use of essential oils for a measurable outcome and is the focus of this women's health clinical aromatherapy nursing and midwifery guide (Buckle 2001). Therapists practicing in women's health will find this to be a useful resource for their practice.

Certified as a clinical aromatherapy practitioner specializing in women's health for 20 years in nursing, I have practiced nursing aromatherapy in the US and UK, have taught nurses, midwives and doulas throughout the US and Chile, developed the first hospital OB unit aromatherapy program in the US and conducted and published research in aromatherapy for postpartum depression.

This book will focus solely on the clinical evidence base— in other words, the results of ethically approved research studies conducted on consenting women (pregnancy/menopause) by nurses, doctors and scientists in clinical environments. The exact essential oils, concentrations and methods will be shared for ease of safe practice with accompanying supportive references. This practical design is a guidebook for busy nurses, midwives and doulas with five minutes to access aromatherapy information for their patients, for the therapist to plan for an upcoming client and any woman interested in proven safe and effective aromatherapy for their health and well-being.

Clinical aromatherapy is a wonderful tool to enhance nursing, midwifery and therapist care of patients and clients, and personal self-care. As a trauma, psychiatric and women's health nurse, I searched for years for this missing component of care.

There is a current explosion of popularity for aromatherapy in the general population with a common belief that "natural = safe" and that one can care for one's family and friends without incurring costly medical bills. Neighbors, family members, clergy, and many well-intentioned and trusted individuals often guide sales and recommendations. Often extreme claims are made without the benefit of formal education in aromatherapy or research studies (evidence base) to support strongly held convictions. Financially, much is to be gained by recommendations of daily use for cures, health and well-being to the tune of millions of dollars.

Women's bodies are miracles, producing miracles and often enduring decades of monthly physical and emotional discomfort. As a woman, nurse, mother and clinical aromatherapist, I've witnessed countless therapeutic benefits from clinical aromatherapy in women's healthcare clinically and personally. As a complementary therapy for practicing nurses and midwives, I'm sharing what I've learned thus far to enhance your practice and encourage you to closely follow the clinical evidence base provided in this book. It has stood the test of time, there's plenty of it and, as the most trusted healthcare professionals, we owe it to the women in our care.

This guidebook serves as a quick hospital, clinic or private practice clinical reference for aromatherapy treatments that have been researched and shown to be safe and effective in various women's healthcare settings. The specific references with a summary of key findings are listed with the individual oils to share with patients, healthcare professionals and skeptical colleagues, and to keep with your aromatherapy supplies.

In pregnancy, this book is a tool for childbirth education as well as a helpful comparison guide for oils and blends brought from home by women for labor and delivery. The section with the largest core clinical evidence base is labor and delivery, offering multiple options for physical and emotional discomforts utilized in midwifery and nursing practice for nearly 30 years. In postpartum care, modern women are seeking gentle options for emotional support in their new role and their family's healthcare. Aromatherapy provides wonderful supportive self-care tools to enhance healing and encourage a woman's journey into motherhood.

In gynecologic (GYN) care, this book can be utilized as a resource to educate and empower teens suffering with painful menstrual cycles, younger women with the physical and emotional misery of premenstrual syndrome (PMS), and midlife women with menopausal havoc, by offering effective, integrative non-pharmaceutical options with few to no side effects.

Nurses and midwives often express frustration with the lack of available quality women's health aromatherapy education, feeling uninformed about which oils are effective, safe or unsafe when their patients inquire about aromatherapy. My sincere hope is that this guide will clarify for the healthcare professional, and the women in their care, the most effective and safest aromatherapy for a wide range of women's health conditions.

As a practitioner, you too can reap the gentle stress-relieving benefits of aromatherapy. In respect to "caring for the caregiver," may this information serve to physically and emotionally support your own self-care and be a health and healing tool for you and your loved ones.

# CHAPTER 1

# What Is Clinical Aromatherapy?

When one thinks of "aroma," one usually thinks of something scented. Images of spas, candles and beach massages come to mind when we hear the term "aromatherapy." In the past decade the world of aromatherapy has experienced phenomenal growth and popularity in the mainstream population outside of the traditional healthcare industry. In 2016, the global aromatherapy market was valued at USD 1.07 billion and is expected to continue to rise in the upcoming years (Grand View Research 2017). This rapid growth in the aromatherapy industry, brought about by profound company loyalty and business opportunities to sell essential oils without any medical background or clinical aromatherapy education, can prove a challenge to the nurse or midwife who is presented with a woman arriving to the hospital in labor with a large bag of blended oils she wants to use. What is safe to use? What will help the woman in labor? The purpose of this book is to provide specific information on essential oils, which can be used to support women's health and to educate the reader/nurses, midwives, doulas and therapists in what we know from aromatherapy research studies on women to inform your clinical practice.

In 2004, the Nobel Prize in Physiology or Medicine was awarded to physiologists Drs Axel and Buck for identifying more than 1000 odor receptors in humans, unraveling the mysteries of our sense of smell and thus highlighting the tremendous therapeutic potential for aromatherapy (Nobel Prize 2004). In my experience, the majority of North American people prefer light floral, citrus or familiar spice scents as an introduction to aromatherapy. We are repelled or warned by unpleasant scents and possess a lifetime of scent memories related to our cultures, traditions and life experiences which all influence our reactions to scent. When possible, particularly in treating emotional conditions, offer your patient a choice of scent, which enhances therapeutic effectiveness.

The tools of aromatherapy are essential oils, steam-distilled or cold-expressed from various parts of aromatic plants. They are very concentrated and, depending on the plant's yield, can be quite expensive. A commonly stated example of the concentration of an essential oil is "Twenty-eight teabags of peppermint herb produce one drop of peppermint essential oil." Very little oil is needed to enjoy the scent or produce a measurable outcome as in clinical aromatherapy.

In hospitals and clinical settings the type of aromatherapy practiced by nurses is known as *clinical aromatherapy*. The difference between mainstream personal aromatherapy and clinical aromatherapy is the educational background of the clinician and clinically evidence-based aromatherapy education specific to clinical areas. Nurses and midwives with advanced education in clinical aromatherapy learn about specific essential oils, their therapeutic properties and methods that have been researched clinically on humans and shown to be effective and safe. Clinical aromatherapy is defined as "the therapeutic use of essential oils for a measurable outcome" (Buckle 2001); in other words, much like a pain scale, we ask the patient their pre- and post-aromatherapy treatment numerical rating for a particular condition. This is known as a Likert scale (0 = no discomfort; 10 = worst discomfort) and is used daily by nurses and midwives in all clinical settings to determine the effects of various treatments.

There are specific essential oils and methods of administration that have been shown in studies (evidence-based) to be effective and safe for particular conditions. Lists of the clinically evidence-based essential oils and methods related to specific conditions will be highlighted throughout the book. The treatments in this book require a maximum of five minutes, which is of utmost importance to a busy clinician.

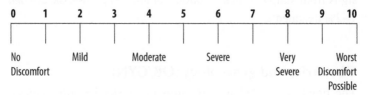

*Likert scale*

## Clinically evidence-based aromatherapy

For this book, we will focus on *clinically evidence-based aromatherapy*, specifically research conducted in approved clinical settings on female subjects (*in vivo*) by healthcare professionals educated in aromatherapy, measuring the before (pre-) and after (post-) effects of an aromatherapy treatment for a particular condition.

We will highlight and focus on the specific *clinical evidence base* for women's health conditions to inform safe and effective nursing and midwifery aromatherapy practice for the OB/GYN aspect of women's healthcare.

## Is there more to aromatherapy than just pleasant scents?

As new scientific studies emerge, surfacing patterns are demonstrating a wide range of physiological and emotional responses before and after clinical aromatherapy treatments. Implementing standardized scales for self-reported physical, emotional and behavioral changes in pain, depression, anxiety and nausea pre- and post-aromatherapy treatments demonstrates statistically significant differences from control groups. Alterations in the hormone and neurotransmitter levels of the neurological and endocrine systems positively correspond to the effects noted on the self-reported scales. This combination of repeated findings offers a glimpse of the future potential for clinical aromatherapy. As we proceed, take note of the number of varied studies indicating positive changes in cortisol, estrogen and serotonin levels and vital signs from simple, quick, economical and very low-risk *external* 1–2% treatments.

## Obstetrics and gynecology (OB/GYN)

The book is divided into sections on obstetrics (pregnancy/ *antenatal or prenatal*, labor and childbirth/ *intrapartum* and after-delivery/ *postpartum*) and gynecology (beginning of menstruation/ *menarche* to end of menstruation/ *menopause*). Each section provides guidance on the most common conditions that have a clinical aromatherapy evidence base. Simple specific guidelines for choosing and preparing aromatherapy treatments related to clinical conditions are given throughout the book. Relevant references are listed alongside the recommendations for quick and easy access to clinical evidence for practice and sharing with colleagues.

My background of 30 years in nursing, 20 woven with hospital and pharmacy clinical aromatherapy practice, program development, consultation and research without any serious complications to mother or baby provides you with an excellent template for safe and effective practice. In select cases a step forward has been the development of simple therapeutic nursing blends of 2–4 single evidence-based oils, thus creating synergies to increase the range of effects and maintain a minimal number of oils to clearly identify positive and negative responses and alter the blend as necessary to obtain a more positive response.

A woman's lifetime hormonal journey can be fairly turbulent physically and emotionally, from menstrual cramps, PMS, pregnancy and menopause; during pregnancy, despite the most perfect birth plan, many obstacles can arise requiring abrupt (and disappointing) changes in direction for the best outcome. Aromatherapy offers women physical and emotional support for multiple OB/GYN conditions and provides the nurse and midwife with safe, gentle, pleasant and effective tools to smooth the rough edges and provide satisfying caring comfort measures.

# Chapter 2

# Methods and Safety

The four methods used in women's health clinical aromatherapy, all of which are external, are the following:

- **Inhalation:** 1–3 drops on a cotton pad or with a personal inhaler (direct), or with a diffuser (indirect). *Quickest route for anxiety, panic, fear, nausea and pain perception.*

- **Skin application/massage:** dilute 1–3 drops essential oils in 5 ml unscented lotion or carrier oil (e.g. grapeseed, jojoba, fractionated coconut). *Best route for any physical pain and discomfort.*

- **Baths (whole body, sitz or foot baths):** add 2–8 drops essential oils to carrier oil for dispersion, then add mix to warm bath water. Don't add to bath during labor. *If time permits, best for insomnia, stress reduction and perineal healing (sitz).*

- **Spritzer:** add oils (12 drops/1 oz bottle) to glass spray bottle, fill with sterile water, shake and spray. Excellent for hot flashes, refreshing for athletes and long days, enhancing the immediate area around women in clinical settings to create their own personal space.

## Preparing a single oil treatment

The normal concentration for a non-pregnant adult is 1–5%, a pregnant woman 0.5–1%, and for labor/postpartum 1–2%.

- 0.5% = 1 drop of essential oil with 10 ml/2 tsp carrier lotion.

- 1% =1 drop of essential oil with 5 ml/1 tsp carrier lotion.

- 2% = 2 drops of essential oil with 5 ml/1 tsp carrier lotion.

- 3% = 3 drops of essential oil with 5 ml/1 tsp carrier lotion.

- 4% = 4 drops of essential oil with 5 ml/1 tsp carrier lotion.

- 5% = 5 drops of essential oil with 5 ml/1 tsp carrier lotion.

As you can see, the amount of carrier lotion, oil, gel or water is always the same, but the number of drops changes to develop your 1–5% percentage. If you need to make it weaker, you add more carrier as in the 0.5% above which would be for pregnancy, young children, the elderly, ill or an individual with a dislike of perceived strong scents.

### If blending more than one oil

First, blend the oils in an empty dropper bottle and label it. It's best to mix the oils together to get a blend of both/all oils and then to add drops of the blend to the carrier lotion, oil, gel or water to give your appropriate concentration (1 drop/5ml = 1%). Alternatively, you can mix oils first in a medicine cup then add the correct amount of carrier lotion or oil to obtain the accurate total percentage.

For example:

1. Mix 3 drops of lavender and 1 drop of lemon together.

2. To make a **1% blend**, you would add 1 drop of this blend to 1 tsp/5 ml of carrier lotion.

3. To make a **2% blend**, add 2 drops/5 ml lotion.

4. In a **2 oz bottle** to make a **1% blend** you add 12 drops total of essential oil blend to 2 oz/60 ml of lotion (1 oz = 30 ml; 2 oz = 60 ml).

5. SHAKE WELL.

6. Always write your blends down.

## Safety

An important aspect of the success with this gentle therapy, particularly with the obstetric patient, is honoring important parameters of safety to maintain as low a risk as possible. Essential oils are strong and very concentrated and therefore only a small amount (i.e. 1–2 drops OB, 1–5 drops GYN) is necessary for a therapeutic outcome.

The degree of concentration and strength of various plant-based remedies is demonstrated in the following diagram, with essential oils shown to be the strongest/most concentrated. When used externally at 1–2% they are a very economical complementary therapy for clinical use.

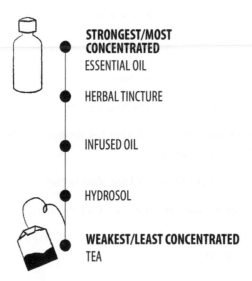

**STRONGEST/MOST CONCENTRATED**
ESSENTIAL OIL

HERBAL TINCTURE

INFUSED OIL

HYDROSOL

**WEAKEST/LEAST CONCENTRATED**
TEA

*A comparison of the strength of various plant-based therapies highlights the concentration of essential oils is the strongest*

All of the clinical evidence has consistently involved external 1–2% applications with rare non-serious side effects that could be the result of the condition, not the aromatherapy. The following is a list of the guidelines that have endured for the past 30 years with thousands of women in hundreds of hospitals on more than three continents and which are recommended for the nurse and midwife to follow.

- Clinically evidence-based education for staff administering aromatherapy.

- All treatments are external (inhalation, skin application, baths and spritzers).

- Only use clinically evidence-based essential oils and methods.

- Essential oils are strong and very concentrated.

- Avoid ingestion.

- Always dilute the essential oils in an unscented white lotion, aloe gel or carrier oil before applying to skin.

- Only 1–2 drops per 5 ml carrier are required for a 1–2% clinical treatment.

- Keep essential oils away from infants, young children, eyes, open wounds and suture lines.

- Keep essential oils in a locked cabinet.

- Always have orifice reducers for droppers in bottles; no wide-mouthed bottles.

- Store in amber or cobalt-blue glass bottles.

- Keep away from sun in a cool, dark cabinet.

- Follow Material Safety Data Sheet (MSDS) for individual essential oils.

- Dispose of oils, bottles and soaked paper towels in double Ziploc bags into hazardous-waste containers.

- Gas chromatography/mass spectrometry (GCMS) analysis for each oil.

## OB precautions

- Avoid essential oils in the first trimester (only lemon inhalation after 10 weeks; Yavari *et al.* 2016).

- Follow current clinical evidence base for safe practice.

- External use only per clinical evidence base.

- Always dilute 0.5–1% until term, 2% labor/postpartum.

- Avoid with epilepsy, high-risk pregnancies, major cardiac, liver or renal disease, preeclampsia, eclampsia, pyrexia, anticoagulant therapy, polyhydramnios, placenta previa, reduced fetal movements, higher multiple pregnancies (Tiran 2016). See key terminology list at the beginning of the book for clarification.

- Exercise caution with twin pregnancies, breech, transverse or unstable fetal position, history of vaginal bleeding, diabetes, asthma, hypertension, hypotension, bleeding disorders, history of miscarriage, hemorrhage, seasonal or multiple allergies to plants, food, aromatics.

- Room spray only with preterm labor.

- Avoid using aromas that the woman dislikes.

## Essential oil safety

- Do not ingest/take essential oils internally.

- Essential oils should not be directly used on to the skin.

- Take care that undiluted essential oils do not come into contact with sensitive areas such as eyes, nose, face, neck.

- Wash hands thoroughly after blending oils or using oils in massage.

- If your hands are sore or cracked, avoid massaging with oils and use gloves when blending oils.

- Keep essential oils away from naked flames: they are highly flammable.

- Keep essential oils away from children.

- Only use essential oil bottles with orifice reducers (internal standard-sized dropper) for each oil when blending.

# Complete list of clinically evidence-based OB/GYN essential oils

| Essential oil | Botanical name | OB/GYN |
|---|---|---|
| Bergamot | *Citrus bergamia* | OB/GYN* |
| Cinnamon | *Cinnamomum zeylancium* | GYN |
| Clary sage | *Salvia sclarea* | OB/GYN |
| Clove | *Syzgium aromaticum* | GYN |
| Cypress | *Cupressus sempervirens* | GYN |
| Eucalyptus | *Eucalyptus globulus* | OB/GYN |
| Frankincense | *Boswellia carterii* | OB/GYN |
| Geranium | *Pelargonium graveolens* | OB/GYN |
| Jasmine | *Jasminum officinale* | OB/GYN |
| Lavender | *Lavandula angustifolia* | OB/GYN* |
| Lemon | *Citrus limon* | OB/GYN* |
| Mandarin | *Citrus reticulata* | OB/GYN |
| Neroli | *Citrus aurantium* | OB/GYN* |
| Peppermint | *Mentha piperita* | OB/GYN |
| Petitgrain | *Citrus aurantium* ssp. *Amara* | OB/GYN* |
| Roman chamomile | *Anthemis nobilis* | OB/GYN |
| Rosemary | *Rosmarinus officinalis* | GYN |
| Rose | *Rosa damascena* | OB/GYN |
| Sweet marjoram | *Origanum marjoram* | GYN |
| Ylang-ylang | *Cananga odorata* | GYN |
| Yuzu | *Citrus junos* | OB/GYN |

\*   *Evidence-based in pregnancy.*

# OBSTETRICS

OBSTETRICS

# CHAPTER 3

# Pregnancy/Prenatal Aromatherapy

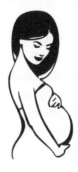

In this chapter we will explore the clinical evidence base for use of aromatherapy during pregnancy: the *prenatal/antenatal* stage. The role of the nurse and midwife as patient advocate and educator is especially important and welcome at this stage. Clinical aromatherapy is practiced in hospitals by nurses and midwives educated in select clinically evidence-based essential oils and methods for measurable therapeutic outcomes.

Given its mainstream popularity, the aromatherapy "industry" is currently worth hundreds of millions of dollars, due to rising healthcare costs, slick and robust marketing from large aromatherapy companies, desire for control of personal and family healthcare and widespread belief that "natural = safe" with perceived minimal risks.

Pregnant women often distrust pharmaceutical companies and are fearful of prescription and over-the-counter medications causing harm to themselves and their developing fetus. Recent survey studies highlighted a wide range of 15–89% of pregnant women admitted to accessing complementary therapies for self-care, with aromatherapy one the most popular. An additional finding is that women rarely informed their healthcare professionals, fearing judgment and lack of healthcare professional knowledge of aromatherapy (Khadivzadeh and Ghabel 2012; Pallivalapila *et al.* 2015; Sibbritt *et al.* 2014).

As a nurse or midwife, the period during pregnancy and childbirth is a perfect time for educating women on the benefits and risks of aromatherapy and complementary therapies alongside childbirth education, dispelling myths of "natural = safe" and developing trust for open dialogue and education. With a captive audience during these nine months, those caring for women enter a sacred space with their patients for promoting physical and emotional self-care as they embark on the unknown journey of pregnancy through early motherhood. This time provides the nurse or midwife with an opportunity to assess mental health history and risks for postpartum depression. Women supporting women is in itself an amazing tool for female well-being.

Pregnancy is a time of significant hormonal upheaval, often leading to multiple physical and emotional discomforts. Many prescription and over-the-counter medications are prohibited during pregnancy due to safety risks. In the early 1960s, the thalidomide tragedy occurred when trusting pregnant women were prescribed a "safe" medication for insomnia, stress and morning sickness/nausea. Thalidomide was ultimately found to be responsible for widespread malformations of infants' limbs, which led to banning the medication; future testing of pharmaceuticals on pregnant women ceased for the next 60 years (Vargesson 2015). In another tragic pharmaceutical story, diethylstilbestrol (DES) was prescribed for pregnant women with morning sickness and led to a significant increased incidence of cervical cancer in their daughters. Fears of pharmaceuticals during pregnancy have increased the popularity of self-care with plant-based remedies (herbs, essential oils, flower essences and nutritional supplements) and various complementary therapies, with the widespread belief that "natural = safe." With concerns about essential oil constituents crossing the placenta and effects on the developing fetus, exercising caution and following the existing evidence base is the recommended route for practice. Due to their immaturity, the fetus's developing immune and detoxification systems are not as effective as those of adults, and are not selective about toxicity. It should therefore be assumed that all essential oils cross the placenta. The essential oil used, its dilution and method of application need to be assessed with regard to risk and potential benefit. The clinical evidence base should be consulted to support the best interest of the woman and fetus, as well as practitioner liability.

This belief of "natural = safe" is often the rationale for exploring aromatherapy during pregnancy and enhances the opportunity for nurses to educate women about the effects on both mother and developing fetus. The importance of open-minded dialogue and strategic assessment questions goes a long way to obtaining vital self-care practices and development of nursing educational tools. Inquiries regarding nutritional and herbal supplement use fit well alongside specific essential oils or blends as well as *methods of use* prior to and during pregnancy.

Most women and those selling oils are unaware that essential oils cross the placenta and can potentially negatively affect fetal growth and development. The risks increase depending on the method of use. The clinical evidence base exclusively concerns *external use* (inhalation, foot baths or skin massage), as absolutely no clinical evidence of internal use with pregnant women exists in any database. According to Tiran, "Essential oils should not be administered orally, vaginally or rectally during pregnancy as the levels that reach the fetus will be excessively high" (2016, p.105). Regarding the development of the fetal brain and spinal cord, Tiran shares that "The blood brain barrier is not well developed in the fetus, allowing substances such as essential oils to reach the central nervous system, which is susceptible to chemical damage"

(2016, p.106). External use at 1–2%, as highlighted in each of the studies, is effective in improving the discomforts of pregnancy with minimal risk to mother or baby. When used externally at 1–2% they are a very economical complementary therapy for clinical use.

During pregnancy, with a myriad of hormonal changes, a woman's sense of smell is often altered, making prior scent preferences and strengths noxious or overpowering and unexpected scents curiously appealing. Offering choices of essential oils from the list at low dilutions of 0.5–1% is amazingly effective, pleasant and extremely safe.

There are currently five clinical aromatherapy studies with pregnant women. Except for lavender, all the oils are from a citrus fruit or plant origin; the oils are lemon, lavender, petitgrain, bergamot and neroli. Of these, lemon essential oil is the only oil that has clinical evidence to support its use in the first trimester, and neroli is the only essential oil that has clinical evidence for use with hospitalized high-risk women. Citrus oils are generally considered the safest oils and, in my clinical experience, are well received, uplifting and effective during pregnancy.

## Pregnancy/prenatal list of clinically evidence-based essential oils

- Bergamot (*Citrus bergamia*)

- Lavender (*Lavandula angustifolia*)

- Lemon (*Citrus limonum*)

- Neroli (*Citrus aurantium var. amara*)

- Petitgrain (*Citrus aurantium*)

## Essential oils for pregnancy

While concerns regarding the adverse effects of prescription and over-the-counter medications lead women toward non-medicinal and herbal alternatives, only five essential oils at 1–2% dilution in select external methods have been studied in clinical settings on pregnant women and shown to be safe and effective.

In the first trimester, often a time of extreme fatigue and nausea, only one essential oil, lemon, is clinically evidence-based (Yavari *et al.* 2014). In the second trimester, a further three studies have examined the effectiveness of lavender, bergamot and petitgrain essential oils (Chen *et al.* 2017; Effati-Darvani *et al.* 2015; Igrarashi 2013). In addition, neroli was studied in the third trimester with high-risk pregnant women (Go and Park 2017). These studies focused on emotional well-being, anxiety, stress, depression and immune support. The importance of maternal stress reduction in pregnancy for the growth and development of the fetus as well as maternal well-being cannot be underestimated.

## Prenatal evidence base
### Bergamot
A distinct citrus scent used to flavor Earl Grey tea.

**Therapeutic properties:** Relaxing and uplifting. Popular oil used for anxiety, depression and stress.

**Method of application:** Inhalation.

**Research:** In Igarashi's (2013) randomized controlled trial, pregnant women were able to select their preferred essential oil from a group of oils high in linalool and linalyl acetate (bergamot, petitgrain and lavender). Inhalation for five minutes with a diffuser improved tension/anxiety and anger/hostility mood scales, and parasympathetic activity increased with observed relaxation. More study is needed to see if these results are repeated.

* ★ Igarashi, T. (2013) "Physical and psychological effects of aromatherapy inhalation on pregnant women: A randomized controlled trial." *Journal of Alternative and Complementary Medicine 19*, 10, 805–810.

## Lavender

A very popular oil with herbaceous and floral scent and a wide range of properties.

**Therapeutic properties:** Calming and soothing, frequently used for stress, anxiety, depression and sleep.

**Method of application:** Inhalation, foot-bath, foot massage.

**Research:** There are three clinical studies which examine the use of lavender in pregnancy. Studies indicated that stress, anxiety and depression scales improved with the use of lavender essential oil; parasympathetic activity also increased, noting observed relaxation with lavender via inhalation, foot-bath or foot massage at 1–2% dilution. Chen *et al.*'s (2017) randomized controlled trial (RCT) showed decreased salivary cortisol and improved IgA (immunoglobulin A) immune function levels in the group that received 70 minutes of aromatherapy massage with lavender essential oil 2% dilution during weeks 16–36.

* Chen, P.J., Chou, C.C., Yang, L., Tsai, Y.L., Chang, Y.C. and Liaw, J.J. (2017) "Effects of aromatherapy massage on pregnant women's stress and immune function: A longitudinal, prospective, randomized controlled trial." *Journal of Alternative and Complementary Medicine 23*, 10, 778–786.

* Effati-Daryani, F., Mohammad-Alizadeh-Charandabi, S., Mirgafourvand, M., Taghizadeh, M. and Mohammadi, A. (2015) "Effect of lavender cream with or without foot-bath on anxiety, stress and depression in pregnancy: A randomized placebo-controlled trial." *Iranian Red Crescent Medical Journal 4*, 1, 63–73.

* Igarashi, T. (2013) "Physical and psychological effects of aromatherapy inhalation on pregnant women: A randomized controlled trial." *Journal of Alternative and Complementary Medicine 19*, 10, 805–810.

## Lemon

The only clinically evidence-based essential oil in the first trimester, lemon has a familiar fresh, crisp citrus scent.

**Therapeutic properties:** Emotionally uplifting with symptoms of depression, helpful for nausea and vomiting, vasoconstrictive support with nosebleeds and varicose veins.

**Method of application:** Inhalation on cotton pad, room diffuser or spritzer.

**Research:** Yavari *et al.* (2014) studied the effectiveness of inhalation of lemon essential oil on nausea. The randomized clinical trial of 100 women in the first trimester concluded that lemon scent could be effective in reducing nausea in pregnancy. Two drops of lemon essential oil diluted in almond oil and inhaled from a cotton pad when nauseated for three minutes, as needed, brought greater relief for nausea and vomiting than without aromatherapy.

* Yavari, K.P., Safajou, F., Shahnazi, M. and Nazemiyeh, H. (2014) "The effect of lemon inhalation aromatherapy on nausea and vomiting of pregnancy: A double-blinded, randomized, controlled clinical trial." *Iranian Red Crescent Medical Journal 16*, 3, e14360.

## Neroli

A floral citrus scent with slight herbaceous notes.

**Therapeutic properties:** Calming for panic and extreme anxiety.

**Method of application:** Inhalation.

**Research:** In Go and Park's (2017) study, hospitalized high-risk pregnant women inhaled neroli for two minutes three times a day for five consecutive days. Improvements were noted in depression, stress and anxiety scores, as well as autonomic nervous systems; changes were all greater in the neroli treatment group than the control group.

★ Go, G.Y. and Park, H. (2017) "Effects of aroma inhalation therapy on stress, anxiety, depression, and the autonomic nervous system in high-risk pregnant women." *Korean Journal of Women Health Nursing 23*, 1, 33–41.

### Petitgrain

Floral, woody scent.

It is much less expensive than neroli with similar properties.

**Therapeutic properties:** Calming and soothing for anxiety and stress, uplifting with depression.

**Method of application:** Inhalation.

**Research:** See the details of Igarashi's (2013) trial under "Bergamot" above.

★ Igarashi, T. (2013) "Physical and psychological effects of aromatherapy inhalation on pregnant women: A randomized controlled trial." *Journal of Alternative and Complementary Medicine 19*, 10, 805–810.

## Clinically evidence-based aroma tips for pregnancy

In addition to traditional nursing assessment and medical history questions, when using aromatherapy it is helpful to ask these questions to determine preferences, allergies or sensitivities:

• Are you allergic to any plants, foods, herbs, spices or scents?

• What are your most positive scent memories/favorite scents?

- What are your most negative scent memories/unpleasant scents?

- What type of remedies do you normally use for headaches, stomach aches, colds, stress or pain?

- In addition to prenatal vitamins, what supplements, herbals, teas or aromatherapy oils do you find helpful? If yes, to herbs or aromatherapy oils: How do you use them?

## First trimester (weeks 10–12)
NAUSEA/MORNING SICKNESS/EMOTIONAL SUPPORT

**Lemon** (*Citrus limon*), the only essential oil clinically studied in the first trimester, can be inhaled, diffused or used with a room spritzer bottle at 1–2% dilution.

Dilute 1 drop of lemon essential oil in 5 ml/1 tsp of water, jojoba or grapeseed oil and inhale for five minutes as needed for nausea and emotional support.

## Second trimester (weeks 13–24)
ANXIETY/DEPRESSION/STRESS/PAIN

**Lavender** (*Lavandula angustifolia*) has been studied more than any other essential oil and tends to be the most popular with women. At 1–2% it can be inhaled on a cotton pad or using a diffuser or spritzer for emotional support and pain relief.

**Lemon** (*Citrus limon*), inhaled on a cotton pad or with a diffuser or room spritzer, is uplifting, antiseptic, decongestant and cheerful.

## Third trimester (25 weeks–term)
PAIN/DEPRESSION/ANXIETY/FEAR

**Bergamot** (*Citrus bergamia*), a beloved citrus scent and well known oil for emotional support, can be inhaled, diffused or used in a spritzer for anxiety, depression, stress and fear.

**Lavender** (*Lavandula angustifolia*) diluted 1% in unscented lotion applied to the area of discomfort or 1% inhalation on a cotton pad often provides pain relief, relaxation and much-needed rest.

**Lemon** (*Citrus limon*), inhaled on a cotton pad or with a diffuser or room spritzer, is uplifting, antiseptic, decongestant and cheerful. It can also be diluted to 1% in aloe gel, lotion or grapeseed oil and applied to skin to soothe varicose veins or applied to fingers to apply pressure to nose to halt nosebleeds.

**Neroli** (*Citrus aurantium*) is a blissful and popular anti-panic and anxiety oil. Dilute 0.5–1% for periodic inhalation with high-anxiety and stressed women.

**Petitgrain** (*Citrus aurantium*), derived from the twigs and leaves of a bitter orange tree, provides emotional balance at 1% inhalation, or used in a diffuser or room spritzer.

# Quick reference table: pregnancy/prenatal

| Condition | Essential oils (blends of 1–3) | Methods* |
|---|---|---|
| Anxiety | Lavender, petitgrain, bergamot, neroli | Inhalation on cotton pad, diffusion, foot-bath, massage 1% after 16 weeks |
| Depression | Lavender, petitgrain, bergamot, lemon, neroli | Inhalation on cotton pad, diffuser, spritzer 1% after 16 weeks |
| Fear | Lavender, neroli | Inhalation on cotton pad or diffuser 1% |
| Hyperemesis | Lemon | Inhalation on cotton pad 1–2% |
| Morning sickness | Lemon | Inhalation on cotton pad 1–2% |
| Pain | Lavender, bergamot | Foot-bath, massage, inhalation on cotton pad 1% |
| Sleep | Lavender, neroli | Foot-bath, inhalation on cotton pad, massage 1% |
| Stress | Lavender, bergamot, petitgrain, lemon | Inhalation on cotton pad, diffuser, foot-bath, massage 1% |

\*    *Adding 1 drop of essential oil to 5ml / 1 tsp lotion or carrier oil creates 1% dilution, the recommended amount during pregnancy.*

CHAPTER 4

# Aromatherapy for Labor and Delivery

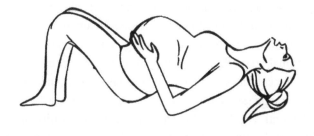

In this chapter we will explore the clinical evidence base for use of aromatherapy during labor and delivery: the *intrapartum* stage. The largest amount of clinical evidence for obstetric (OB) aromatherapy exists during the intrapartum period once a woman is in established term labor. In 1990, at a large referral hospital in Oxford, England, averaging 6000 births a year, a team of midwives instituted an eight-year aromatherapy study of 8058 women in labor and delivery (Burns *et al.* 2000). With an aromatherapist's knowledge and expertise, they selected ten essential oils with therapeutic properties for anxiety, nausea, pain and potential to augment contractions in dysfunctional labor. Their list of ten clinical study oils, which are still used in labor and delivery today, were lavender, mandarin, lemon, frankincense, Roman chamomile, eucalyptus, peppermint, clary sage, rose and jasmine. Over the past 30 years nurses and midwives in the US, UK and Chile have followed the clinical evidence base of these ten oils and methods without one single serious incident to mother or baby. Only mild side effects (i.e. headache, nausea and rash) were experienced by 1% of the women. The duration, numbers of women, safety and effectiveness of aromatherapy treatments in labor and delivery make a strong case for this clinically evidence-based program to be the healthcare standard for nursing and midwifery practice.

This chapter will highlight these ten essential oils, their various uses and the data collected from women receiving these nursing and midwifery aromatherapy treatments. Essential oils possess multiple chemical constituents and therefore have many therapeutic properties and clinical indications. Lavender alone has antiseptic, analgesic, sedative and skin-healing properties and is clinically indicated for pain, anxiety, sleep and skin healing. As clinical aromatherapy increases globally, we are now seeing additional research studies and adding to the clinical evidence base. Recent labor studies with bergamot, geranium, neroli and sweet orange essential oils have increased our list to 14.

Several US State Boards of Nursing require proof of education for nurses practicing complementary therapies such as aromatherapy, the most popular therapy with women. Public trust is very high for nurses in part because of the licensure requirement that proves that the necessary education and knowledge base has been obtained to practice safely and competently. Aromatherapy is not part of standard nursing or midwifery university education and requires the individual to complete the education on his or her own. Unfortunately, courses are not always readily available or institutionally funded. With 30 years of safe and effective nursing and midwifery clinical aromatherapy practice for women, this begs the question: Why would nurses practice outside of the evidence base? However, due to widespread exposure outside the healthcare realm, clinical course availability, the cost of education and a belief that because it is natural it is safe—or "our oils are pure" so none of the previous knowledge applies—that's exactly what is emerging. It is hoped that following the information provided and the ease of use will inspire nurses and midwives in clinical settings to follow the evidence-based essential oils and methods for labor and delivery, ignore far-fetched claims and, when possible, attend clinical aromatherapy courses.

The majority of prescription pharmaceuticals and over-the-counter medications are considered off limits for pregnant woman, leaving few options for illness or the discomforts of pregnancy. Fear and mistrust of the pharmaceutical industry has led women toward alternative choices of remedies for their discomforts often outside the traditional healthcare realm. A recent troubling US trend of exaggerated claims for essential oil products, made by sales representatives without proof of clinical evidence, has led to safety issues for pregnant women and infants. Product sales training rather than professional education has led to a vast increase in incident reports ranging from essential oil oversensitivity and skin burns to uterine hyperstimulation and respiratory distress in infants. Women in labor arriving at the hospital with hidden bags of blended oils are an all too common occurrence. Often a belief in "natural is safe," alongside significant trust in a friend, family or clergy with an entrenched belief system and promise of significant financial gain, is challenging for healthcare professionals to navigate. Significant conflict may also exist for the nurse or midwife without evidence-based aromatherapy education to provide wise counsel about appropriate use and safety concerns: a perfect storm.

As these trends continue to cause concern, I recommend a potential solution to protect our patients. As we've done in nursing for decades to avoid misuse or accidental overmedication, send personal aromatherapy oils home or lock them up with valuables for safekeeping. This provides an opportunity for education on the evidence-based aromatherapy policy, choices, education of staff and standard of practice for their utmost safety. They can still receive aromatherapy and save their oils for future use. By following the clinically evidence-based lists in this book, the nurse or midwife is equipped with essential oil and method lists and supportive references for their practice as well as patient educational tools. Comparison of the list of clinically evidence-based oils used exclusively in your program can be made with the patient's kit to enhance mutual understanding of safe and effective clinical use of essential oils. Sharing with your patient the provided list of clinically evidence-based oils and methods is an educational starting point for you and your patient.

The majority of women are fearful of the pain of labor and experience a range of anxiety from "butterflies in the stomach" to full-blown panic and hysteria. In an anxious state, muscles contract, the heart rate increases, breathing is shallow, as all of our systems experience a "fight or flight" response. Studies and nursing experience have shown that inhalation of select essential oils quickly decreases the unpleasant experience of anxiety and fear by slowing the release of stress hormones. A relaxed woman has a greater likelihood of experiencing a shorter and more comfortable labor experience. With simple inhalation of relaxing essential oils, breathing slows, muscles relax, vital signs improve and women report lessened feelings of anxiety and fear, thus allowing the natural process of labor to unfold.

Labor is an ideal time to introduce aromatherapy by experientially laying the foundation for physical and emotional comfort measures into early motherhood. Almost 12,000 additional women in labor have received aromatherapy treatments in the US, UK and Chile, guided by the clinical evidence base from the studies by Burns *et al.* (2000, 2007), with close to 9000 women without a single serious issue to mother or baby over a 30-year period. Following the clinical evidence base provides a strong, safe and effective foundation for the nurse, midwife and doula at the bedside. The eight-year study of 8058 women in Oxford (Burns *et al.* 2000) who received midwifery clinical aromatherapy treatments during childbirth demonstrated the successful integration of a complementary therapy for anxiety, pain, nausea and improved contractions which we have copied in hospitals in the US and Chile since 2008. The study highlighted the effectiveness and safety of the controlled use of ten selected essential oils in specific methods, to achieve measurable therapeutic results such as decreasing the use of opioids (pethidine/Demerol) in the aromatherapy group for the study duration from 6% to 0.2%. An additional RCT study by the same researcher (Burns *et al.* 2007) with more than 500 women in Italy, using five of the initial ten oils, reinforced the effectiveness and safety of these oils and methods, with fewer infants (0 vs. 6) from the aromatherapy group mothers than control group mothers needing to be transferred to the neonatal intensive care unit (NICU). It is possible that relaxing the mother with aromatherapy during labor and childbirth decreased stress on the fetus, leading to fewer NICU admissions.

Since 2008, these studies of selected essential oils and methods have been the foundation of my women's health clinical aromatherapy nursing and midwifery courses and hospital programs in the US and Chile.

Our nursing program's recent data from more than 550 women in labor highlights the most effective essential oils and percentage of improvement with simple aromatherapy treatments for pain, anxiety, nausea and contractions. In all of our clinical programs, we use a 0–10 Likert scale (0 = no pain; 10 = worst pain), as is customary in nursing for measuring patients' pain levels. The patient is asked to rate their particular condition (i.e. anxiety, pain, nausea, grief and contractions) prior (pre) to aromatherapy treatment and then to rate again 10–30 minutes (post) aromatherapy treatment. The following graphs share the pre- and post-data of the top four most effective essential oils for anxiety, pain and contractions with women in labor as well as the overall percentage improvement for ease of interpretation.

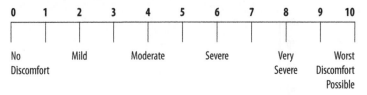

*Likert scale*

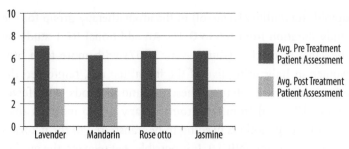

*Pre-/post-treatment labor anxiety*

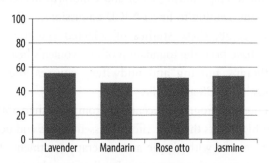

*Percentage improvement in labor anxiety*

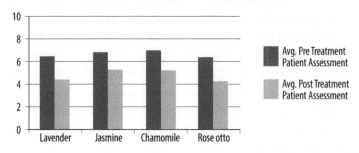

*Pre-/post-treatment labor pain*

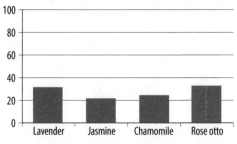

*Percentage improvement in labor pain*

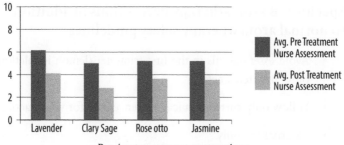

*Pre-/post-treatment contractions*

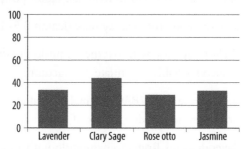

*Percentage improvement in progression of contractions*

It is important to highlight the fact that aromatherapy is not for everyone. Always respect a woman's personal choice and belief system, and be mindful of conditions that prohibit safe use of aromatherapy (i.e. benefit vs. risk).

There is a middle road between "all or nothing" to avoid disappointing a woman determined to have an aromatic childbirth experience, such as a room spritzer rather than direct application, or a massage with unscented carrier lotion to provide caring comfort without risks. Often, due to a changing clinical scenario in labor, aromatherapy may be best left for the less acute postpartum period. In our experience, women appreciate knowing that the opportunity is not completely lost and that aromatherapy will still be available for them.

## Specific OB aromatherapy precautions in addition to normal aromatherapy safety guidelines

- Avoid essential oils in the first trimester (lemon inhalation only, after ten weeks).

- Follow only current clinical evidence base for safe practice.

- External use only.

- Always dilute 0.5–1% until term, 2% labor/postpartum.

- For preterm labor, room spray only (lemon 0.5–1%).

- Avoid clary sage use with oxytocin infusion (induction) as it can uncomfortably potentiate contractions.

- Avoid clary sage with VBAC (vaginal birth after cesarean) or any prior uterine scar due to risk of uterine rupture.

- Use lavender and Roman chamomile with caution with asthma and seasonal allergies.

- Avoid use of clary sage or lavender (sedative hypotensive oils) with epidural until blood pressure normalizes post-epidural.

- Avoid rose with increased bleeding or hemorrhage.

- Use frankincense with caution where there is a prior history of psychosis or thought disorder.

- Avoid aromatherapy with epilepsy, high-risk pregnancies, major cardiac, liver or renal disease, preeclampsia, eclampsia, pyrexia, anticoagulant therapy, polyhydramnios, placenta previa, reduced fetal movements, higher multiple pregnancies (Tiran 2016).

- Exercise extra caution with twin pregnancies, breech, transverse or unstable fetal position, history of vaginal bleeding, diabetes, asthma, allergies, hypertension, hypotension, bleeding disorders, history of miscarriage, hemorrhage, seasonal or multiple allergies to plants, foods or aromatics.

- Discontinue aromatherapy in a medical emergency or rapid change in maternal or fetal status.

## Specific guidelines

- Essential oils should always be used in the correct dosage.

- Nurses and midwives who are pregnant should also follow pregnancy guidelines regarding the use of essential oils.

- Complete an assessment/checklist sheet prior to using essential oils. Consult criteria for selection, contraindications, and methods of use.

- Document pre- and post-aromatherapy treatment evaluation.

- Nurses and midwives practicing aromatherapy clinically should have successfully completed clinically evidence-based education on OB/GYN essential oils.

- Do not use essential oils on infants under three months of age.

- Avoid peppermint and eucalyptus oils around or in contact with infants.

## Labor and delivery list of clinically evidence-based essential oils

- Bergamot (*Citrus bergamia*)

- Clary sage (*Salvia sclarea*)

- Eucalyptus (*Eucalyptus globulus*)

- Frankincense (*Boswellia carterii*)

- Geranium (*Pelargonium graveolens*)

- Jasmine (*Jasminum grandiflorum or Jasminum sambac*)

- Lavender (*Lavandula angustifolia*)

- Lemon (*Citrus limonum*)

- Mandarin (*Citrus reticulata*)

- Neroli (*Citrus aurantium var. amara*)

- Peppermint (*Mentha piperita*)

- Roman chamomile (*Anthemis nobilis*)

- Rose (*Rosa damascena*)

- Sweet orange (*Citrus sinensis*)

## Essential oils for labor and delivery (*intrapartum*)
### Bergamot (*Citrus bergamia*)
A distinct citrus scent used to flavor Earl Grey tea.

**Therapeutic properties:** Bergamot is a popular oil used for anxiety, depression and stress. It is a light, fresh, uplifting oil for winter blues, anxiety and depression.

**Method of application:** Massage, inhalation.

**Research:** In Dhany *et al.*'s (2012) study of 2158 women, bergamot and frankincense were the most popular oils (1350 women) of the seven tested, with inhalation and massage being the most common methods of using them. Findings were that general, spinal and epidural anesthetic rates were significantly less in the aromatherapy group than the control group.

★ Dhany, A.L., Mitchell, T. and Foy, C. (2012) "Aromatherapy and massage intrapartum service impact on use of analgesia and anesthesia in women in labor: A retrospective case note analysis." *Journal of Alternative and Complementary Medicine 18*, 10, 932–938.

## Clary sage (Salvia sclarea)

Strong herbaceous, musky, sage-like scent.

**Therapeutic properties:** Clary sage is an extremely relaxing, euphoric, antispasmodic and analgesic oil, making it ideal for labor. It has been shown in studies and in our data to enhance uterine contractions while relieving uterine pain.

**Safety:** Avoid use with VBAC or with any prior uterine scar to decrease risk of uterine rupture.

Avoid use with pitocin infusion as clary sage can uncomfortably potentiate contractions causing hyperstimulation.

Because of its hypotensive properties, allow blood pressure to normalize post-epidural for 30–60 minutes before using or repeating. Avoid use if patient is hypotensive.

Identified as phytoestrogenic, thus contraindicated during pregnancy and for people with history of reproductive system cancers.

**Method of application:** Massage, inhalation.

**Research:** Burns *et al.* (2000) indicated that clary sage was used by 87% for augmenting contractions; 70% in dysfunctional labor did not require oxytocin infusion and 92% had standard vaginal deliveries (SVD). At the beginning of the eight-year study, 13% of women who used aromatherapy also used opioids (pethidine/Demerol) for pain control. By the end of the study the opioid use in the aromatherapy group was 0.2%. In light of the current opioid epidemic, aromatherapy offers safe, effective, nonaddictive options for pain control. Overall, fewer women using aromatherapy required induction and progressed to SVD than in the control groups. Burns *et al.* (2007) indicated that clary sage was used by 11% of the women, with fewer overall NICU admissions in the aromatherapy group (0) compared with the control group (6). In Lee and Hur's (2011) study, clary sage was combined in a massage blend used by partners/spouses with lavender, frankincense and neroli; labor pain and anxiety were significantly reduced. Dhany *et al.* (2012) demonstrated significantly lower rates of use of spinal and general anesthetics overall with the aromatherapy group; 10% of the women were treated with clary sage.

★   Burns, E., Zobbi, V., Panzeri, D., Oskrochi, R. and Regalia, A. (2007) "Aromatherapy in childbirth: A pilot randomized controlled trial." *BJOG 114*, 7, 838–844.

★   Burns, E.E., Blamey, C., Ersser, S.J., Barnetson, L. and Lloyd, A.J. (2000) "An investigation into the use of aromatherapy in intrapartum midwifery practice." *Journal of Alternative and Complementary Medicine 6*, 2, 141–147.

★   Dhany, A.L., Mitchell, T. and Foy, C. (2012) "Aromatherapy and massage intrapartum service impact on use of analgesia and anesthesia in women in labor: A retrospective case note analysis." *Journal of Alternative and Complementary Medicine 18*, 10, 932–938.

★   Lee, M.K. and Hur, M.H. (2011) "Effects of the spouse's aromatherapy massage on labor pain, anxiety and childbirth satisfaction for laboring women." *Korean Journal of Women Health Nursing 17*, 3, 195–204.

## *Eucalyptus (Eucalyptus globulus)*

Strong medicinal menthol scent.

**Therapeutic properties:** An aid for congestion and upper respiratory infections. Inhalations on cotton pad for easing congestion are often appreciated. It is an uplifting room refresher during the winter months and long labors.

**Safety:** Avoid use with general anesthetic as it has been noted potentially to enhance clearing of barbiturates (1.8 cineole).

Avoid around infants, as with peppermint, to decrease risk of respiratory distress.

**Method of application:** Inhalation.

**Research:** Rated by women in labor as the top oil for enhancing well-being and as a decongestant for upper respiratory infections.

* ★ Burns, E.E., Blamey, C., Ersser, S.J., Barnetson, L. and Lloyd, A.J. (2000) "An investigation into the use of aromatherapy in intrapartum midwifery practice." *Journal of Alternative and Complementary Medicine 6*, 2, 141–147.

## *Frankincense (Boswellia carterii)*

Sweet, resinous scent. Slows and calms anxiety, panic and the rapid breathing of anxiety and grief. Soothes respiratory infections and bronchial irritation. Enhances spiritual and meditative practice.

**Therapeutic properties:** Frankincense is extremely calming for anxiety, panic and hysteria during labor. It is supportive as a grief and spiritual aid in fetal demise and the complex emotions arising from adoption, loss and guilt. One or two drops inhaled on a cotton pad can be used for panic and hysteria. Blend with lemon and/or rose for grief and spiritual support.

**Method of application:** Inhalation, massage.

**Research:** In the studies, frankincense was used by inhalation for anxiety and fear and in massage for pain. In Burns *et al.*'s (2000) study it was rated in the top 2–3 of the most helpful essential oils for both pain and anxiety. In our clinical programs, frankincense is exceptional for panic and hysteria-type anxiety, as well as grief support. In Lee and Hur's (2011) study, in which frankincense was combined in a massage blend that was used in massage by partners/spouses with lavender, clary sage and neroli, labor pain and anxiety were significantly reduced.

★ Burns, E., Zobbi, V., Panzeri, D., Oskrochi, R. and Regalia, A. (2007) "Aromatherapy in childbirth: A pilot randomized controlled trial." *BJOG 114*, 7, 838–844.

★ Burns, E.E., Blamey, C., Ersser, S.J., Barnetson, L. and Lloyd, A.J. (2000) "An investigation into the use of aromatherapy in intrapartum midwifery practice." *Journal of Alternative and Complementary Medicine 6*, 2, 141–147.

★ Dhany, A.L., Mitchell, T. and Foy, C. (2012) "Aromatherapy and massage intrapartum service impact on use of analgesia and anesthesia in women in labor: A retrospective case note analysis." *Journal of Alternative and Complementary Medicine 18*, 10, 932–938.

★ Lee, M.K. and Hur, M.H. (2011) "Effects of the spouse's aromatherapy massage on labor pain, anxiety and childbirth satisfaction for laboring women." *Korean Journal of Women Health Nursing 17*, 3, 195–204.

## Geranium (Pelargonium graveolens)

Geranium is a strong, floral, warming, uplifting and balancing oil.

**Therapeutic properties:** Geranium is wonderful for edema and fluid retention by stimulating the lymphatic system. Its strong floral scent is best softened with lemon for younger women. Spritzers with lemon and geranium refresh, uplift and stimulate the room and mood. For edematous lower extremities, blend in lotion with mandarin for gentle upward ankle and calf massage. Its powerful aroma will tend to override other oils; use small amounts in blends.

**Method of application:** Inhalation, massage, diffusion.

**Research:** Rashidi-Fakari *et al.* (2015) indicated a significant decrease in self-reported anxiety with the State-Trait Anxiety Inventory (STAI), a standardized tool to measure anxiety pre- and post-treatments, and noted reduction in diastolic blood pressure with inhalation during the first stage of labor. In Tansvisuit *et al.* (2017), diffusion reduced pain in latent and early active labor.

* Rashidi-Fakari, F.R., Tabatabaeichehr, M., Kamali, H., Rashidi-Fakari, F. and Naseri, M. (2015) "Effect of inhalation of aroma of geranium essence on anxiety and physiological parameters during first stage of labor in nulliparous women: A randomized clinical trial." *Journal of Caring Sciences 4*, 2, 135–141.

* Tanvisut, R., Kuntharee, T. and Theera, T. (2017) "Efficacy of aromatherapy for reducing pain during labor: A randomized controlled trial." *Archives of Gynecology and Obstetrics 297*, 5, 1145–1150.

## Jasmine (*Jasminum grandiflorum or Jasminium sambac*)
Exotic floral scent.

**Therapeutic properties:** Provides strength and fortitude to the laboring woman while enhancing contractions and the process of labor. Antidepressive and helpful for severe anxiety; produces a feeling of inner strength and has an energizing effect on the emotions. Builds confidence.

Anecdotally, in multiple clinical cases, jasmine diluted 2% in a lower abdominal massage enhanced difficult third-stage placental delivery. Its antidepressant properties provide emotional support and confidence with postpartum depression. A uniquely useful essential oil physically and emotionally.

**Method of application:** Massage, inhalation, diffusion.

**Research:** In Tanvisut *et al.* (2017), jasmine by diffusion was selected by women in labor 2–5 times more often for pain than the other essential oil choices, and overall pain scores in latent and early active labor were significantly lower than in the control group. In Dhany *et al.* (2012), 15% of women chose jasmine, and they noted an overall significantly lower use of anesthetics; as an analgesic massaged into the lower abdomen, the pain scores overall were lower in latent and early active labor but not in late active labor.

★ Burns, E.E., Blamey, C., Ersser, S.J., Barnetson, L. and Lloyd, A.J. (2000) "An investigation into the use of aromatherapy in intrapartum midwifery practice." *Journal of Alternative and Complementary Medicine 6*, 2, 141–147.

★ Dhany, A.L., Mitchell, T. and Foy, C. (2012) "Aromatherapy and massage intrapartum service impact on use of analgesia and anesthesia in women in labor: A retrospective case note analysis." *Journal of Alternative and Complementary Medicine 18*, 10, 932–938.

★ Tanvisut, R., Kuntharee, T. and Theera, T. (2017) "Efficacy of aromatherapy for reducing pain during labor: A randomized controlled trial." *Archives of Gynecology and Obstetrics 297*, 5, 1145–1150.

## Lavender (Lavandula augustifolia)

Floral herbal scent.

Lavender is the most widely used and studied of all essential oils. Its wide range of therapeutic properties, ready availability and low cost make it very useful for *all* clinical programs and especially during labor and childbirth. If your clinical program can only support a small range of essential oils, *always* include lavender. Keep in mind that, due to its widespread popularity, many women automatically choose lavender over all others when offered a list of essential oils. It is usually a good fit; however, due to seasonal allergies or asthma, another choice may be preferable at times.

**Therapeutic properties:** The therapeutic properties of lavender range from sedative to analgesic, making it a wonderful oil to calm anxiety, ease labor pain and headaches, and provide periods of rest during labor. In early labor, inhaling one drop on a cotton pad calms the mother and support person, and enhances a relaxed, therapeutic environment.

May accelerate labor by relaxing the mother.

Lavender is a very diverse oil for physical and emotional conditions, and is thus highly recommended as a component of any clinical program. Blend lavender and rose for a labor massage, as well as emotional support for anxiety and depression.

**Method of application:** Inhalation, massage.

**Research:** In the following studies, the methods of use for lavender (*Lavandula angustifolia*) were inhalation and massage (skin application). In Burns *et al.*'s (2000) large eight-year study of 8058 women in the UK, lavender was used more than any other oil for anxiety and pain, with both conditions showing greater than 50% improvement, contributing to less use of epidural pain relief and significant decreased use of opioid (pethidine/Demerol) pain medication in the aromatherapy group from 13% at the start of the study to 0.2% seven years later. In Burns *et al.*'s (2007) randomized controlled trial of 531 women in Italy, lavender was the most frequently used oil (38%), with pain the most common symptom treated, followed by anxiety; the study noted the decrease in pain perception with those treated for anxiety. Significant to this study were the numbers of NICU transfers: none in the aromatherapy group and six in the control group. In Abbaspoor and Mohammadkani's (2013) study of 60 women, there were interesting findings of significantly decreased pain intensity and shorter duration of first and second stages of labor in the lavender group compared with the control group. Lavender was viewed by midwives and women who received treatments as a viable non-pharmacological, simple, inexpensive and effective option for pain, fear and anxiety, with noted effects of shortened labor and positive neonatal outcomes.

Findings indicate that lavender was very effective to varying degrees for pain, fear and anxiety during labor and it was often the most popular choice for clinical studies and patient choice. All studies were single oil, apart from Lee and Hur (2011), which used a massage blend with lavender, clary sage, frankincense and neroli applied by the birth partner for ten minutes every hour from 5 cm dilation onward, which significantly improved labor pain and anxiety.

* Abbaspoor, Z. and Mohammadkhani, S.L. (2013) "Lavender aromatherapy massages in reducing labor pain and duration of labor: A randomized controlled trial." *African Journal of Pharmacy and Pharmacology 7*, 8, 426–430.

* Burns, E., Zobbi, V., Panzeri, D., Oskrochi, R. and Regalia, A. (2007) "Aromatherapy in childbirth: A pilot randomized controlled trial." *BJOG 114*, 7, 838–844.

* Burns, E.E., Blamey, C., Ersser, S.J., Barnetson, L. and Lloyd, A.J. (2000) "An investigation into the use of aromatherapy in intrapartum midwifery practice." *Journal of Alternative and Complementary Medicine 6*, 2, 141–147.

* Dhany, A.L., Mitchell, T. and Foy, C. (2012) "Aromatherapy and massage intrapartum service impact on use of analgesia and anesthesia in women in labor: A retrospective case note analysis." *Journal of Alternative and Complementary Medicine 18*, 10, 932–938.

* Lee, M.K. and Hur, M.H. (2011) "Effects of the spouse's aromatherapy massage on labor pain, anxiety and childbirth satisfaction for laboring women." *Korean Journal of Women Health Nursing 17*, 3, 195–204.

* Tanvisut, R., Kuntharee, T. and Theera, T. (2017) "Efficacy of aromatherapy for reducing pain during labor: A randomized controlled trial." *Archives of Gynecology and Obstetrics 297*, 5, 1145–1150.

* Yazdkhasti, M. and Pirak, A. (2016) "The effect of aromatherapy with lavender essence on severity of labor pain and duration of labor in primiparous women." *Complementary Therapies in Clinical Practice 25*, 81–86.

## Lemon (Citrus limonum)

Fresh, bright citrus.

**Therapeutic properties:** Inhalation eases mild nausea, colds and upper respiratory infections, and a spritzer is physically refreshing and emotionally uplifting during a long labor. Lemon's vasoconstrictive properties work well applied topically 2% for a nosebleed or to ease the heaviness of varicose veins. It is often used to enhance the effect of other oils. A drop of lemon added to lavender, rose, frankincense or jasmine lifts the overall scent, softening them and improving their appeal.

**Method of application:** Inhalation.

**Research:** In Yavari *et al.*'s (2014) prenatal study, Lemon was found to be helpful for nausea via inhalation. Burns *et al.* (2000) found it to be uplifting and to enhance feelings of overall well-being. In our programs, it is useful as an additional option for nausea, in uplifting and refreshing long labor, and in grief blends.

* Burns, E.E., Blamey, C., Ersser, S.J., Barnetson, L. and Lloyd, A.J. (2000) "An investigation into the use of aromatherapy in intrapartum midwifery practice." *Journal of Alternative and Complementary Medicine 6*, 2, 141–147.

## Mandarin (Citrus reticulata)

Sweet and citrusy.

**Therapeutic properties:** Women find it (alone or with lemon) to be uplifting and gently calming for agitation, restlessness, nervous tension and insomnia. As an abdominal massage, mandarin eases digestive upsets, bloating and flatulence, and gentle upwards lower-leg and ankle massage (alone or with geranium) eases edematous lower legs and ankles. Often used to enhance the effect of other oils. Cheerful and uplifting, mandarin is known as the gentlest and safest essential oil, making it perfect during labor and childbirth.

**Method of application:** Inhalation.

**Research:** In Burns *et al.*'s (2007) study conducted in Italy, mandarin was the second most common oil (after lavender) of five oils selected by women primarily for anxiety and fear. In this study, there were fewer NICU admissions with the aromatherapy group (0 vs. 6 in the control group) and labor duration was shortened. Mothers rated it as calming and enhancing for overall well-being. Interestingly, in Burns *et al.*'s (2000) study conducted in the UK with ten essential oils, it was not one of the top oils selected, possibly due to cultural preferences.

* Burns, E., Zobbi, V., Panzeri, D., Oskrochi, R. and Regalia, A. (2007) "Aromatherapy in childbirth: A pilot randomized controlled trial." *BJOG 114*, 7, 838–844.

* Burns, E.E., Blamey, C., Ersser, S.J., Barnetson, L. and Lloyd, A.J. (2000) "An investigation into the use of aromatherapy in intrapartum midwifery practice." *Journal of Alternative and Complementary Medicine 6*, 2, 141–147.

## Neroli (Citrus aurantium)
An uplifting sweet, citrusy, floral scent.

**Therapeutic properties:** Neroli can be inhaled alone or used with sweet orange, mandarin and/or lemon in a room spritzer to freshen and uplift. Helpful for heightened anxiety, panic and fear.

**Method of application:** Inhalation, spritzer.

**Research:** In Namazi *et al.* (2014), anxiety scores decreased significantly more at dilations 3–4 cm and 6–8 cm in the neroli group compared with the control group, with diluted neroli on a gauze pad attached to women's gowns and changed every 30 minutes throughout labor progression. In Lee and Hur's (2011) study, a spousal massage with a blend of neroli, lavender, frankincense and clary sage significantly reduced labor pain and anxiety scores.

* Lee, M.K. and Hur, M.H. (2011) "Effects of the spouse's aromatherapy massage on labor pain, anxiety and childbirth satisfaction for laboring women." *Korean Journal of Women Health Nursing 17*, 3, 195–204.

* Namazi, M., Amir Ali Akbaria, S., Mojab, F., Talebi, A., Alavi Majd, H. and Jannesari, S. (2014) "Aromatherapy with citrus aurantium oil and anxiety during the first stage of labor." *Iranian Red Crescent Medical Journal 16*, 6, e18371.

## Peppermint (Mentha piperita)
Familiar, cool and minty.

**Therapeutic properties:** Excellent essential oil for easing nausea during transition, post-op and with migraine headaches. Peppermint's analgesic properties ease headache and back pain. Refreshing during long labors.

**Safety:** Always keep away from infants and young children under three years of age due to reported respiratory distress with peppermint exposure in this age group. For skin sensitivity issues, it is best to dilute in lotion to 1% (1 drop/5 ml lotion) before applying to skin.

**Method of application:** Inhalation.

**Research:** In Burns *et al.*'s (2000) study, inhalation of peppermint for nausea and vomiting was chosen by 96% of 1149 women, rating improvement at 50%. Peppermint was the highest rated overall by patients for nausea and vomiting.

★ Burns, E.E., Blamey, C., Ersser, S.J., Barnetson, L. and Lloyd, A.J. (2000) "An investigation into the use of aromatherapy in intrapartum midwifery practice." *Journal of Alternative and Complementary Medicine* 6, 2, 141–147.

★ Dhany, A.L., Mitchell, T. and Foy, C. (2012) "Aromatherapy and massage intrapartum service impact on use of analgesia and anesthesia in women in labor: A retrospective case note analysis." *Journal of Alternative and Complementary Medicine* *18*, 10, 932–938.

## Roman chamomile (Authemis nobilis)

Herbal grassy scent.

**Therapeutic properties:** The most antispasmodic essential oil, Roman chamomile provides wonderful support for muscular and abdominal cramping and pain in labor. It is anti-inflammatory and good for skin rashes, eczema and itching. It is also calming and supportive for periods of rest and sleep. Blend with clary sage and lavender for labor pain.

**Safety:** Caution should be taken with seasonal allergies, hay fever and asthma due to its relationship to ragweed.

**Method of application:** Massage.

**Research:** The main finding in the two studies by Burns *et al.* (2000, 2007) suggests that two essential oils, clary sage and Roman chamomile, were effective in alleviating pain; the use of opioids decreased significantly in the aromatherapy group from the beginning to the end of the eight-year study (Burns *et al.* 2000). In the author's private practice and clinical programs, multiple aromatherapy treatments using Roman chamomile alone or in pain blends for muscle, labor and menstrual cramps have been very effective.

★   Burns, E., Zobbi, V., Panzeri, D., Oskrochi, R. and Regalia, A. (2007) "Aromatherapy in childbirth: A pilot randomized controlled trial." *BJOG 114*, 7, 838–844.

★   Burns, E.E., Blamey, C., Ersser, S.J., Barnetson, L. and Lloyd, A.J. (2000) "An investigation into the use of aromatherapy in intrapartum midwifery practice." *Journal of Alternative and Complementary Medicine 6*, 2, 141–147.

## Rose (Rosa damascena)

Strong, sweet, floral.

**Therapeutic properties:** Eases stress and anxiety while enhancing the natural process of labor. Luxurious floral scent supports women at risk for or with prior history of postpartum depression, and provides grief support. It is luxurious blended with lavender for inhalation or labor massage for emotional support. It is thought to help tone the uterus. Known as the "queen of flowers," this delicate, feminine oil is very popular and effective for labor and childbirth. Very expensive and very little needed, so use sparingly.

**Safety:** Avoid with excessive bleeding or hemorrhage.

**Method of application:** Inhalation, foot-bath, massage.

**Research:** Rose was rated in Burns *et al.* (2000) as the most effective oil for calming anxiety by mothers during labor. Kheirkhah *et al.* (2014), using inhalation and foot-bath, noted significant reduction in anxiety in the first stage of labor compared with the control group.

★   Burns, E.E., Blamey, C., Ersser, S.J., Barnetson, L. and Lloyd, A.J. (2000) "An investigation into the use of aromatherapy in intrapartum midwifery practice." *Journal of Alternative and Complementary Medicine 6*, 2, 141–147.

* Dhany, A.L., Mitchell, T. and Foy, C. (2012) "Aromatherapy and massage intrapartum service impact on use of analgesia and anesthesia in women in labor: A retrospective case note analysis." *Journal of Alternative and Complementary Medicine 18*, 10, 932–938.

* Kheirkhah, M., Vali Pour, N.S., Nisani, L. and Haghani, H. (2014) "Comparing the effects of aromatherapy with rose oils and warm foot bath on anxiety in the first stage of labor in nulliparous women." *Iranian Red Crescent Medical Journal 16*, 9, e14455.

## Sweet orange (*Citrus sinensis*)

Familiar citrus scent.

**Therapeutic properties:** Cheerful and uplifting for depression and anxiety in room diffuser or cotton pad inhalation. Sweet orange has been shown to decrease self-reported anxiety in labor with no significant changes noted in physiological parameters (blood pressure, pulse and respiration).

**Method of application:** Inhalation, diffuser.

**Research:** Rashidi-Fakari *et al.*'s (2015) study showed greater reduction in anxiety among the group of women who had been exposed to orange essential oil than the control group.

* Rashidi-Fakari, F., Tabatabaeichehr, M. and Mortazavi, H. (2015) "The effect of aromatherapy by essential oil of orange on anxiety during labor: A randomized clinical trial." *Iranian Journal of Nursing and Midwifery Research 20*, 6, 661–664.

# Methods of use during labor (1–2% blends)
## Inhalation

1–2 drops of undiluted essential oil onto a cotton pad for brief nausea, panic and intense congestion;

may attach to a gown for 10 minutes and repeat every 2 hours. With ongoing stress, blues, depression or nausea dilute to 2% on a cotton pad and directly inhale as needed. *Do not use this method for asthmatics.*

## Massage/skin application

Best for pain, any physical discomfort, labor support.

Add two drops of essential oil or blend to 5 ml unscented lotion or grapeseed carrier oil. A maximum of three oils may be used in a blend (e.g. add 1 drop each of 3 different essential oils to 15ml grapeseed carrier oil).

## Foot-bath

Best for early labor, warmth, hygiene and emotional support.

Fill foot-bath with warm water, blend 4–6 drops of essential oil into carrier oil (for improved dispersion in water) then add to bath. Soak feet for a minimum of 10–15 minutes.

## Personal diffuser

Indirect subtle environment enhancement.

Add 1–2 drops of essential oil or blend to the filter of a cold air fan diffuser. Use only for 10 minutes in each half hour.

## Spritzer/spray bottle

Best for uplifting environment, decreasing stress and infection control.

Add 4–6 drops of essential oils to empty glass spray bottle, then fill to neck with sterile or distilled water. Shake well and spray around room near the mother, avoiding eyes.

## Labor methods

Undiluted inhalation with just 1–2 drops on a cotton pad held or attached to gown for acute panic, hysteria, extreme congestion, unrelenting nausea and grief (Burns *et al.* 2000, 2007; Dhany *et al.* 2012). Otherwise, 2% on a cotton pad for ongoing use with nausea, anxiety, stress and depression.

All body/skin applications (massage, sprays) are 1% pregnancy, 2% labor-postpartum and oils are first diluted in carrier oil before adding to the bath so they'll mix with water.

## Clinically evidence-based aroma tips for labor

### Early labor arrival with anxiety and fear

Have the woman choose one out of a selection of four familiar calming and uplifting oils (e.g. lavender, lemon, mandarin, sweet orange). Put a couple of drops on a cotton pad for her to inhale as a welcome and to calm her fear and anxiety.

### Increasing anxiety, slow progression of labor

Foot-bath with 4–6 drops of 2% rose or lavender oil. This provides dual benefits of inhaling the scent and skin absorption, and also teaches her body the calming properties of the oils for later reference.

### Epidural, fear of needles

Use 1–2 drops of 2% rose blend on a cotton pad, instructing her to take slow deep breaths to distract and calm her while the needle is inserted.

### Labor progressing, increasing discomfort

Jasmine or lavender 2% in lotion massaged into lower back and/ or abdomen.

### Long labor or heavy energy

Make a personal room spritzer with sweet orange and lemon 2% and spray around room to lightly freshen room and uplift energy.

### Nausea and indigestion

Inhalations of 2% peppermint, lemon or mandarin, according to personal preference. If one doesn't work, try another until she finds the best one.

### Nosebleed

Apply 2% lemon to the bridge of the nose and squeeze for ten minutes or until bleeding stops. Repeat as needed.

### Headache

Lavender 2% in lotion, inhaled and gently massaged on temples, forehead, back of neck and temperomandibular joint (TMJ) area. For migraine headache with nausea, inhale peppermint 1% together with lavender massage.

### Lower-leg and ankle edema

Foot-bath with 2% geranium, and upwards massage from ankle to knee with geranium and mandarin 2% in lotion as needed for skin tightness, discomfort and swelling.

### Rest and sleep

Use lavender and/or mandarin 2% for shoulder massage, inhalation on cotton pad or sheet spritzer.

## Enhance contractions

Use clary sage and/or rose 2% in lotion to massage lower abdomen and around wrists and ankles. Avoid clary sage with pitocin as it can potentiate contractions and increase discomfort. Avoid clary sage with preterm labor, VBAC or any prior uterine scar.

Visualization exercise: Offer a cotton pad with 2 drops of rose oil and encourage the woman to close her eyes and visualize a rose bud slowly opening to full bloom.

## Back labor pain

Blend jasmine and lavender or clary sage and Roman chamomile 2% in lotion and firmly massage into the lower back from the natural waist to the sacrum to ease discomfort. Apply firm counter-pressure to sacrum during contraction. Also, warm baths are comforting while inhaling the oil via cotton pad, room spray or diffuser; adding oil to the water risks eye contact with infant and is best avoided.

## Leg cramps

Use Roman chamomile alone or with lavender 2% in lotion to massage into lower legs and any areas of cramping.

## Exhaustion

Use geranium and lemon in a diffuser, bowl of warm water or spritzer to freshen the room and uplift the woman and supporters.

## Hysteria, extreme anxiety, panic and/or screaming

Frankincense inhalation on cotton pad, fastened to gown or spritzer around upper body, avoiding eyes. If possible, encourage slow, deep breaths.

## Depression

If there is a prior history or current risk of depression, choose oils during labor that can extend through postpartum to support emotional health. Jasmine, rose, lavender and bergamot are all good choices to offer and to alternate through the days ahead. Observe her response for any positive sign such as a smile or pleasant memory to inform the choice.

## Grief

Frankincense and rose softened with lemon or mandarin in a spritzer have been very helpful for the anxiety, stress and profound grief of a fetal demise/"stillbirth." Encouraging the mother to spray around herself alone or with her partner/spouse provides a sacred space for them while the therapeutic properties of the essential oils soften the emotional pain, providing the mother necessary strength. Spritzing the blanket that the parents hold the baby in has proven to be an extremely beneficial tool, decreasing their anxiety and fear.

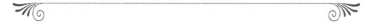

Thoughtful attention toward supporting women physically and emotionally with clinically evidence-based aromatherapy in labor and delivery paves the way toward enhanced postpartum comfort and well-being. In addition, we are introducing tools and demonstrating self-care for early motherhood and beyond. Many women have shared with me how powerful it is when the nurse gives them permission to continue to focus on caring for themselves as well as their infant. The role of nurses and midwives with the new mother is extremely influential, and clinical aromatherapy conveys the message that she's important and deserves the personal care.

## Quick reference table: labor and delivery

The choices remind the practitioner that there are multiple oils that are effective for each condition. Give the patient a choice. If it doesn't work, try another until she has a positive response. Also, note cultural preferences as we have found that essential oils related to positive, comforting memories and experiences can be more effective.

| Condition | Essential oils (blends of 1–3) | Methods |
|---|---|---|
| Anxiety, stress and tension | Lavender, rose, frankincense, mandarin, neroli, clary sage, Roman chamomile, geranium, bergamot | Inhalation on cotton pad, diffuser, hand or shoulder massage |
| Backache/back labor | Clary sage, lavender, Roman chamomile, jasmine | Massage lower back with lotion blend |
| Congestion | Eucalyptus, peppermint, lemon, frankincense | Inhalation on cotton pad or inhaler |
| Depression | Lavender, rose, jasmine, geranium, bergamot, mandarin, lemon, sweet orange | Inhalation on cotton pad, spritzer and/or diffuser |
| Edema | Geranium, mandarin | Upward massage from ankle to knee with lotion blend |
| Grief | Rose, frankincense, lavender, mandarin | Spritzer, diffuser, inhalation on cotton pad |
| Hyperventilating, panic | Frankincense, lavender, neroli, rose | Inhalation on cotton pad |
| Insomnia | Lavender, mandarin, Roman chamomile, neroli | Inhalation on cotton pad, shoulder massage, spritzer on sheets, diffuser |
| Nausea and vomiting | Peppermint, mandarin, lemon | Inhalation on cotton pad |

| | | |
|---|---|---|
| Pain (labor) | Roman chamomile, clary sage, lavender, jasmine, frankincense | Inhalation on cotton pad and massage to lower abdomen and back with lotion blend |
| Refresh and restore/energize | Lemon, peppermint, geranium, eucalyptus, bergamot | Inhalation on cotton pad, diffuser or spritzer |
| Dysfunctional or stalled labor, contractions | Clary sage, rose, lavender | Massage lower abdomen and around ankles, inhalation on cotton pad |
| Swollen perineum | Lavender | Sitz baths with 2% diluted in carrier oil, then add to bath |
| Uplift/well-being | Lemon, eucalyptus, peppermint | Inhalation on cotton pad, spritzer, diffuser |

Chapter 5

# Postpartum Aromatherapy

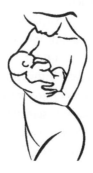

The postpartum period is an important time as the woman embarks on the sacred and overwhelming journey of motherhood. Focus quickly shifts from the pregnant woman to the baby, which can be met with the new mother's concealed mixed emotions, along with physical discomforts and altered body image. By gently relaxing the new postpartum mother, aromatherapy opens emotional pathways while teaching her the pleasure and simplicity of aromatic self-care. Physically and emotionally, she is on an unfamiliar rollercoaster with a sore, leaking body, important new role, shifting hormones and lots of advice. Her need for nursing and midwifery care is critical at this point and the rewards are immense and will be remembered for her lifetime. In multiple studies (Afshar *et al.* 2015; Hadi and

Hanid 2011; Kianpour *et al.* 2016; Metawie *et al.* 2013; Olapour *et al.* 2013), simple inhalations of lavender alone or with rose oil (Conrad and Adams 2012) have been shown to decrease anxiety, stress, blues and pain perception, while affording the exhausted new mother much-deserved rest. As hormone levels shift 2–3 days after delivery, many women are emotional, often sad and tearful; the "baby blues" are normal and last less than two weeks. Especially important during this limited time with the new mother is evaluating previous history of and risk factors for postpartum depression which can guide the choice for specific essential oils. Wei *et al.* (2008) found a total rate of major and minor postpartum depression for all cultures at greater than 25% or one in every four women.

Many women in the postpartum stage are young and healthy, without medical conditions or routine pharmaceutical medication, thus slipping under the radar of healthcare professionals' potential screening for developing concealed emotional conditions. In a culture with mental health stigmas, the lack of routine depression screening reinforces a woman's inclination to conceal her true emotional state, fearing she'll be labeled as emotionally unstable. Ongoing dialogue and screening throughout pregnancy regarding emotional health would identify high-risk women and foster an environment of communication to share her feelings and concerns. Screening is definitely encouraged for all women during pregnancy, with a postpartum follow-up to improve psychological care and services.

The all too common result of the negative stigma surrounding mental health issues and concern regarding safety of prescription medication during lactation is that many women suffer in silence and self-treat with various remedies. Studies indicate that close to 50% of college-educated women experiment with some form of complementary alternative medicine, with aromatherapy rated as one of the most popular (Eisenberg *et al.* 1998).

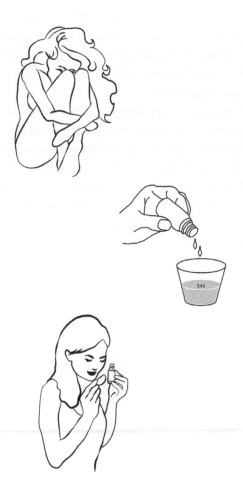

Our nursing and midwifery data from more than 200 postpartum women indicate that simple aromatherapy inhalations and massages improve anxiety and depression up to 63%. In our postpartum depression and anxiety aromatherapy research study (Conrad and Adams 2012), it was anecdotally noted that one-third of the group with postpartum depression had a prior history of depression even as distant as ten years prior to this pregnancy and of duration as short as six months. Identifying woman at risk as early as possible provides an opportunity for early detection, education and tools such as aromatherapy for self-care. The patient can complete simple, standardized questionnaires such as the globally recognized Edinburgh Postpartum Depression Scale (EPDS) and Generalized Anxiety Disorder (GAD7) in ten minutes and reveal important psychological risk factors.

Aromatherapy as a complementary therapy alongside orthodox medical treatment has been shown to improve depression and anxiety more rapidly and to a greater degree than medical treatment alone (Conrad and Adams 2012). Our clinical aromatherapy postpartum anxiety and depression study considered results after four weeks of twice-weekly ten-minute aromatherapy treatments (inhalation or hand massage) with 2% lavender and rose essential oils.

The following two graphs demonstrate the results of the aromatherapy treatments at four weeks for depression and anxiety after a total of eight ten-minute treatments.

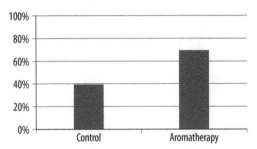

*Anxiety: GAD7 score improvements after 4 weeks*

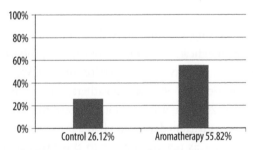

*Depression: EPDS score improvements after 4 weeks*

In addition, our nursing and midwifery hospital program's recent data from more than 500 postpartum women highlight the most effective essential oils and percentage of improvement with simple aromatherapy treatments for anxiety, pain, nausea and grief.

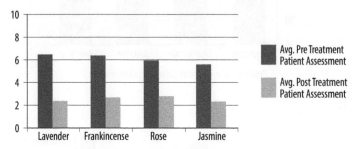

*Postpartum pre-/post-treatment anxiety scores*

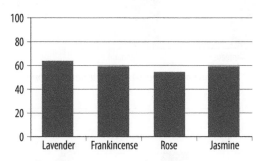

*Postpartum percent anxiety improvements*

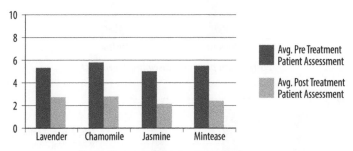

*Postpartum pre-/post-treatment pain scores*

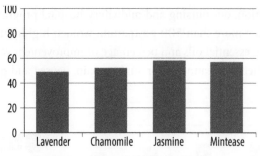

*Postpartum percent pain improvements*

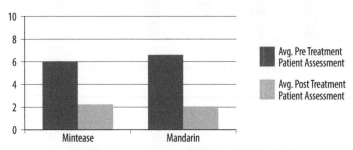

*Postpartum pre-/post-treatment nausea scores*

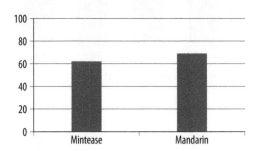

*Postpartum percent nausea improvements*

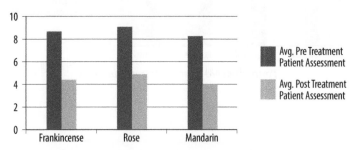

*Postpartum pre-/post-treatment grief scores*

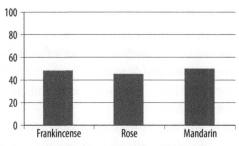

*Postpartum percent grief improvements*

## Postpartum essential oil evidence base

The evidence base for the postpartum period consists of essential oils predominately for support of the newly delivered mother's physical comfort, emotional well-being and enhancement of lactation. Special considerations and precautions for both the mother and infant bring special attention to this stage. Stress reduction measures such as aromatherapy improve healing, enhance lactation and encourage smoother transitions to motherhood. When possible, educate the new mother in the various therapeutic oils and methods for her while reinforcing limited infant exposure.

The pure strength of essential oils can overpower newborns' delicate developing systems so caution with exposure is warranted. Recommendations are to delay infant exposure until 3–6 months of age and at that point only as needed for conditions unrelieved by gentler, less concentrated measures. Always avoid exposure to peppermint and strong menthol essential oils with infants due to their immature respiratory systems.

On several occasions nurse midwives in my courses have shared cases of neonatal respiratory distress related to mothers self-treating with essential oils during labor and delivery. These mysterious scenarios led the nurse midwives to further their own education in maternity aromatherapy. Upon further investigation by the nurse midwives with the mothers about what oils were used, they discovered that the oil in common in all cases of neonatal respiratory distress had been peppermint alone or in blends. As I continue to share these incidents in class, frequently a nurse or midwife will share a similar case in their practice, always related to peppermint use by the mother near the infant, which they've previously been uncomfortable to share due to denial by mothers or staff fervent in the belief that their essential oils are "pure" and thus could not cause harm.

This issue would benefit from open and honest professional dialogue and education followed by inclusion in childbirth education with future parents. On our hospital postpartum units, it is our policy and practice for safety to avoid use of peppermint oil and eucalyptus near infants. When a mother is nauseated or has a migraine headache and prefers peppermint or eucalyptus, she is instructed to avoid topical application and only use it by direct inhalation on a cotton pad when the infant is not in the room, removing the pad from the room and washing her hands before holding her infant. Lemon and mandarin are effective alternatives for nausea and lavender for pain, so offering these options may remove any risks as well as provide education for future options. It is futile to be negative about a particular brand of essential oils; nursing and midwifery education is best focused on essential oils and methods that have been studied and for which evidence exists for their effectiveness and safety in the clinical realm.

## Postpartum list of clinically evidence-based essential oils

- Fennel (*Foeniculum vulgare*)

- Jasmine (*Jasminum grandiflorum or Jasminium sambac*)

- Lavender (*Lavandula angustifolia*)

- Neroli (*Citrus aurantium var. amara*)

- Rose (*Rosa damascena*)

- Sweet orange (*Citrus sinensis*)

- Ylang-ylang (*Cananga odorata*)

- Yuzu (*Citrus junos*)

## Essential oils for postpartum care
### *Fennel (Foeniculum vulgare)*
Sweet, spicy anise-like scent.

**Therapeutic properties:** Supportive for digestion, fluid retention, lactation and expectorant. Phytoestrogenic properties, so contraindicated during pregnancy and with reproductive cancer history.

**Methods of application:** Massage, inhalation, diffusion.

**Research:** In Agustina *et al.* (2016), fennel (and jasmine) in a diffuser and aromatherapy massage decreased cortisol levels and significantly increased breast milk production. In Mikaningtyas *et al.* (2017), special lacta massage using fennel essential oil increased prolactin levels and breast milk production. According to Mikaningtyas *et al.*, "During the lactation process, there are two hormones that play an important role in maintaining the lactation process, namely the hormone prolactin to increase the production of breast milk and hormone oxytocin which cause the secretion of breastmilk."

- ★ Agustina, C., Hadi, H. and Widyawati, M.N. (2016) "Aromatherapy Massage as an Alternative in Reducing Cortisol Level and enhancing Breastmilk Production on Primiparous Postpartum Women in Semarang." *Asian Academic Society International Conference.*

- ★ Mikaningtyas, E. *et al.* (2017) "Lacta Massage using Fennel Essential oil to increase Prolactin Hormone Levels in Postpartum Mothers." *International Journal of Science and Research.*

## *Jasmine (Jasminum grandiflorum or Jasminium sambac)*
Exotic floral scent.

**Therapeutic properties:** Reduces stress in the postpartum woman, helpful for blues and depression with an energizing and strengthening effect on the emotions. Builds confidence.

**Methods of application:** Massage, inhalation, diffusion.

**Research:** In Agustina *et al.* (2016), jasmine (and fennel) in a diffuser and aromatherapy massage decreased cortisol levels and significantly increased breast milk production.

> ★ Agustina, C., Hadi, H. and Widyawati, M.N. (2016) "Aromatherapy Massage as an Alternative in Reducing Cortisol Level and enhancing Breastmilk Production on Primiparous Postpartum Women in Semarang." *Asian Academic Society International Conference.*

## *Lavender (Lavandula angustifolia)*
Fresh, herbal, floral scent.

**Therapeutic properties:** In postpartum care, a lavender drop on a cotton pad for inhalation or hand massage is a gift to a new mother to decrease the fear, anxiety or depression often associated with her new role as mother as well as providing much-deserved sleep. Antiseptic, antibacterial, sedative and analgesic; the perfect all-round oil for pain, anxiety, sleep and healing.

**Methods of application:** Inhalation, massage, sitz bath.

**Research:** Afshar *et al.* (2015) demonstrated that lavender 10% inhalations (ten deep breaths on cotton balls in a cylinder) four times a week for eight weeks showed significant improvement in sleep quality compared with the control group. Vakilian *et al.* (2011) compared lavender sitz baths using 5–7 drops twice a day for ten days, showing significantly less redness of the perineum in the lavender group than the povidone iodine group, with fewer experiencing pain after ten days. Olapour *et al.* (2013) noted improved pain control, decreased heart rate and greater patient satisfaction than the control group, with five-minute inhalations of 10% lavender at four, eight and 12 hours post-op cesarean, and recommended lavender as a multimodal (not sole) analgesic post-op cesarean. Kianpour *et al.* (2016) noted that utilizing inhalations of lavender every eight hours for four weeks resulted in significant improvement, greater than control groups, with stress, anxiety and depression scales at two-week, one- and three-month evaluations. Conrad and Adams' (2012) blend of 2% lavender and rose inhalations or hand massages for ten minutes twice a week for four weeks significantly improved GAD7 anxiety and EPDS depression scores at two weeks, with greater improvement at four weeks. Imura *et al.*'s (2006) most interesting finding indicated that one aromatherapy massage on day one or two, in addition to improving mood, enhanced mother–infant interactions and thus bonding. Agustie *et al.* (2017) recommend specialty oxytocin massage combined with lavender post c-section for statistically increased prolactin levels and increased production of breast milk.

★ Afshar, M.K., Moghadam, Z.B., Taghizadeh, Z., Bekhradi, R., Montazeri, A. and Mokhtari, P. (2015) "Lavender fragrance essential oil and the quality of sleep in postpartum women." *Iranian Red Crescent Medical Journal 17*, 4, e25880.

★ Agustie, P.R. *et al.* (2017) "Effect of oxytocin massage using lavender essential oil on prolactin level and breast milk production in primiparous mothers after caesarean delivery." *Belitung Nursing Journal 3*, 4, 337–344.

★ Asazawa, A.D., Kato, Y., Yamaguchi, A. and Inoue, A. (2017) "The effect of aromatherapy treatment on fatigue and relaxation for mothers during the early puerperal period in Japan: A pilot study." *International Journal of Community Based Nursing and Midwifery 5*, 4, 365–375.

★   Conrad, P. and Adams, C. (2012) "The effects of clinical aromatherapy for anxiety and depression in the high-risk postpartum woman—A pilot study." *Complementary Therapies in Clinical Practice 18*, 3, 164–168.

★   Hadi, N. and Hanid, A.A. (2011) "Lavender essence for post-cesarean pain." *Pakistan Journal of Biological Sciences 14*, 11, 664–667.

★   Imura, M., Misao, H. and Ushijima, H. (2006) "The psychological effects of aromatherapy-massage in healthy postpartum mothers." *Journal of Midwifery and Women's Health 51*, 2, e21–27.

★   Kianpour, M., Mansouri, A., Mehrabi, T. and Asghari, G. (2016) "Effect of lavender scent inhalation on prevention of stress, anxiety and depression in the postpartum period." *Iranian Journal of Nursing and Midwifery Research 21*, 2, 197–201.

★   Lee, S.O. and Hwang, J.H. (2011) "Effects of aroma inhalation method on subjective quality of sleep, state anxiety, and depression in mothers following cesarean section delivery." *Journal of Korean Academy of Fundamentals of Nursing 18*, 1, 54.

★   Metawie, M.A.H., Amasha, H.A., Abdraboo, R.A. and Ali, S.A. (2013) "Effectiveness of aromatherapy with lavender oil in relieving post caesarean incision pain." *Journal of Surgery 3*, 2–1, 8–13.

★   Olapour, A., Behaeen, K., Akhondzadeh, R., Soltani, F., al Sadat Razavi, F. and Bekhradi, R. (2013) "The effect of inhalation of aromatherapy blend containing lavender essential oil on cesarean postoperative pain." *Anesthesiology and Pain Medicine 3*, 1, 203–207.

★ Vakilian, K., Atarha, M., Bekhradi, R. and Charman, R. (2011) "Healing advantages of lavender essential oil during episiotomy recovery: A clinical trial." *Complementary Therapies in Clinical Practice 17*, 1, 50–53.

★ Vaziri, F., Shiravani, M., Najib, F.S., Pourahmad, S., Salehi, A. and Yazdanpanahi, Z. (2017) "Effect of lavender oil aroma in the early hours of postpartum period on maternal pains, fatigue, and mood: A randomized clinical trial." *International Journal of Preventive Medicine, 8*, 29.

## *Neroli (Citrus aurantium)*

Uplifting light sweet floral scent.

**Therapeutic properties:** Especially supportive as an inhalation with anxiety, fear and panic. Enhances slower breathing and focus if hyperventilating. Appreciated by anxious young women.

**Method of application:** Massage.

**Research:** In Imura *et al.*'s (2006) study, neroli combined with lavender in aromatherapy massage improved postpartum mothers' physical and mental status and improved ratings for mother–infant interactions.

★ Imura, M., Misao, H. and Ushijima, H. (2006) "The psychological effects of aromatherapy-massage in healthy postpartum mothers." *Journal of Midwifery and Women's Health 51*, 2, e21–27.

## *Rose (Rosa damascena)*

Strong, sweet, floral.

**Therapeutic properties:** Rose calms anxiety, soothes grief and has a balancing effect on the hormonal system, all perfect for the postpartum woman!

**Method of application:** Inhalation, massage.

**Research:** Conrad and Adams' (2012) pilot study demonstrated that either inhalation on a cotton pad or hand massage with rose and lavender 2% ten minutes twice weekly for four weeks decreased anxiety (GAD7) and depression (EPDS) scores more significantly compared with the control group, measured again at two and four weeks, with progressively greater improvements noted. Of special note with regard to methodology, statistically significant improvements for the EPDS depression scale were almost identical for the two methods, with inhalation 55.46% and hand massage 56.28% improvement (control group 26.12%).

* Conrad, P. and Adams, C. (2012) "The effects of clinical aromatherapy for anxiety and depression in the high-risk postpartum woman—A pilot study." *Complementary Therapies in Clinical Practice 18*, 3, 164–168.

## Sweet orange (Citrus sinensis)

Full sweet citrus scent.

**Therapeutic properties:** Cheerful, familiar and calming, this is a good choice during winter months and with individuals opposed to floral and herbal scents.

**Method of application:** Massage.

**Research:** In Asazawa *et al.*'s (2017) study, each postpartum woman received one 20-minute hand and forearm massage on days 1–7 with one of five diluted essential oils. Self-reported fatigue decreased and relaxation score improved significantly with sweet orange and yuzu.

★ Asazawa, A.D., Kato, Y., Yamaguchi, A. and Inoue, A. (2017) "The effect of aromatherapy treatment on fatigue and relaxation for mothers during the early puerperal period in Japan: A pilot study." *International Journal of Community Based Nursing and Midwifery 5*, 4, 365–375.

## Ylang-ylang *(Cananga odorata)*

Exotic, potent, sweet floral scent.

**Therapeutic properties:** Demonstrated support with hypertension and tachycardia from anxiety and fear. Wonderful choice for irritability and anger issues. It is clinically noted to be best at 1–2% alone or blended; any stronger causes headaches!

**Method of application:** Massage.

**Research:** In Asazawa *et al.*'s (2017) study, each postpartum woman received one 20-minute hand and forearm massage on days 1–7 with one of five diluted essential oils. Self-reported fatigue decreased and relaxation score improved significantly with all oils, and most significantly with sweet orange and yuzu.

★ Asazawa, A.D., Kato, Y., Yamaguchi, A. and Inoue, A. (2017) "The effect of aromatherapy treatment on fatigue and relaxation for mothers during the early puerperal period in Japan: A pilot study." *International Journal of Community Based Nursing and Midwifery 5*, 4, 365–375.

## Yuzu *(Citrus junos)*

Fresh, soft, floral scent.

**Therapeutic properties:** Uplifting welcome option for anxiety, depression and overall well-being.

**Method of application:** Massage.

**Research:** In Asazawa *et al.*'s (2017) study, each postpartum woman received one 20-minute hand and forearm massage on days 1–7 with one of five diluted essential oils. Self-reported fatigue decreased and relaxation score improved significantly with sweet orange and yuzu.

★   Asazawa, A.D., Kato, Y., Yamaguchi, A. and Inoue, A. (2017) "The effect of aromatherapy treatment on fatigue and relaxation for mothers during the early puerperal period in Japan: A pilot study." *International Journal of Community Based Nursing and Midwifery 5*, 4, 365–375.

## Clinically evidence-based aroma tips for postpartum care

### Celebrate the mother

A luxurious lotion blend of lavender 3 drops, jasmine 2 drops and rose lotion 1 drop in 10ml of lotion as a hand or shoulder massage is a wonderful way to congratulate the new mother and celebrate the miracle she's just accomplished. In addition, the therapeutic properties of the essential oils are emotionally supportive and balancing as her hormonal levels begin to shift.

### Rest and sleep

Lavender spritzer on pillow, inhalation on cotton pad or shoulder massage with lavender 2% in lotion relaxes the body and mind for much-needed rest.

### Baby blues

Room spritzer with sweet orange 10 drops, neroli 2 drops and ylang-ylang 1 drop in 1 oz sterile water in a glass spray bottle.

## Abdominal pain and cramping
Lavender 12 drops diluted in 1 oz lotion and massaged into lower abdomen eases discomfort and promotes rest.

## C-section pain
Lavender inhalation on a cotton pad and 2% lotion as above, staying at least 2 inches away from suture line, is relaxing, thus decreasing muscle tension and post-op discomfort.

## Increased lactation/breast milk production
Inhalation on a cotton pad, or diffuser or massage with diluted 2% jasmine, lavender or fennel.

## Anxiety and stress
Inhalation on cotton pad with rose, neroli, lavender or ylang-ylang 2% alone or blend of any two..

## Depression
Inhalation on a cotton pad with 2% rose and lavender or jasmine or sweet orange and neroli. Check her preference for floral or citrus scents, offering her a choice and alternating throughout her stay to determine the best combination. In my experience, culture influences scent preference and ultimately the effectiveness.

## Elevated blood pressure
Inhalation or hand massage with 2% ylang-ylang and lavender for 10 minutes, checking blood pressure before and after treatment. May repeat once after 30 minutes.

### Sore perineum

Lavender 2% in grapeseed oil added to warm sitz baths soaking for 15 minutes two times a day for three days after vaginal birth to ease perineal discomfort and support skin and tissue healing.

### Grief

Rose or frankincense 1–2 drops inhalation on a cotton pad.

The postpartum nurse and midwife are in an opportune position to provide supportive care and invaluable experiential tools and education for self-care. Nurses' and midwives' encouragement of postpartum women, giving them permission to make time to care for themselves with aromatherapy, exercise, quiet time and good nutrition, goes a long way toward reducing future guilt, martyrdom and resentment. This was consistent feedback received during our postpartum study as the women were required to receive treatments unaccompanied, subliminally giving them the message that self-care was important for themselves and their new role as mother.

# Quick reference table: postpartum care

| Condition | Essential oils (blends of 1–3) | Methods |
|---|---|---|
| Anxiety | Rose, lavender, neroli, ylang-ylang, sweet orange, jasmine | Inhalation on cotton pad |
| Baby blues | Rose, jasmine, lavender, sweet orange, neroli | Inhalation on cotton pad, shoulder or hand massage, spritzer |
| Depression | Rose, jasmine, lavender, neroli, sweet orange | Inhalation on cotton pad or inhaler, spritzer, diffuser, massage, bath |
| Edema | Geranium, fennel | Upward massage in lotion |
| Fatigue | Sweet orange, lavender | Inhalation on cotton pad, diffuser, spritzer |
| Grief | Rose, lavender | Spritzer, inhalation on cotton pad |
| Insomnia | Lavender, neroli | Inhalation on cotton pad, spritzer on sheets |
| Lactation | Jasmine, fennel, lavender | Inhalation on cotton pad, massage, diffuser |
| Nausea | Lavender, sweet orange | Inhalation on cotton pad |
| Pain | Lavender, jasmine | Massage area of discomfort, avoid suture line |
| Stress | Lavender, rose, neroli, ylang-ylang, fennel, jasmine | Inhalation on cotton pad, shoulder or hand massage |

# GYNECOLOGY

Studies estimate that globally between 80 and 97% of women experience at least one physical or psychological symptom related to their menstrual cycle in their reproductive years (Halbreich 2003; Ju *et al.* 2014; Milewicz and Jedrzejuk 2006; Wittchen *et al.* 2002). In 2002, the preliminary findings of the Women's Health Initiative (WHI) multicenter trial indicated significant increases in cardiac, stroke and cancer risks for women taking hormone replacement therapy (HRT) which led to prematurely discontinuing the study. This was followed by popular pharmaceuticals for pain and depression revealing serious previously unknown risk factors, leading to overall mistrust of standard medical treatments for women's physical and emotional health. Lack of trust in the medical community and specifically the pharmaceutical industry has led women to access complementary therapies, particularly for hormonal and emotional conditions, without sharing their use with their healthcare professional. The focus of taking sole responsibility for one's own health has altered the relationship between women and their healthcare providers both positively and negatively. Nurses and midwives are in perfect positions of trust and accessibility to educate and assess complementary and alternative medicine (CAM) use, especially herbal and nutritional supplementation and essential oils, which all have potential to interact with medical conditions and pharmacological treatments.

During routine assessments, some or all of the following questions may provide information on personal use:

- Do you use any remedies that you find helpful?

- Have you tried massage, aromatherapy, acupuncture, herbal medicine?

- What makes you feel better/helps the most?

- What do you find gives you the best relief for menstrual cramps, PMS, hot flashes, insomnia, etc.?

- In addition to over-the-counter or prescription medications, what herbals, supplements or oils do you choose to use for your premenstrual, menstrual or menopausal discomforts?

- Have you ever tried any herbals, supplements or essential oils?

- Do you take them internally or externally?

- How much and how often?

- What oils or herbs are in the blend?

- Could we look at the ingredients of the blend together?

Opening dialogue with women establishes your role as educator, caregiver and trusted patient advocate. Trust has shifted outside of the medical realm, and although personal responsibility is important, well-intentioned lay people without formal education or qualifications are often the ones informing our patients about aromatherapy and supplementation.

As we shift to intriguing advances in the field of psycho-neuroendocrinology and clinical aromatherapy, the potential for application in women's health is emerging, which also highlights the need for continued research.

Interesting scientific developments are emerging in the field of clinical aromatherapy through the combination of individuals' subjective responses and measurements of pre- and post-treatment stress, hormone and neurotransmitter levels. In multiple aromatherapy studies, specific stress, depression and female reproductive hormone and neurotransmitter levels (cortisol, serotonin and estrogen) improved alongside women self-reporting improvement of PMS, menstrual and menopausal discomforts. These were all accomplished with inhalation or massage treatments with various single essential oils (rose, lavender, yuzu, bergamot, neroli). When the level of the "stress hormone" cortisol decreases, the "anti-depressant neurotransmitter" serotonin increases, estrogen levels are balanced, symptoms of depression improve and feelings of well-being are enhanced. We are seeing all of these changes with simple aromatherapy treatments. Studies have shown (Rapkin and Akopians 2012) that lowered serotonin levels correlate with a rise in PMS symptoms. With aromatherapy treatments that improve serotonin levels administered only in the luteal phase, when PMS symptoms are most prevalent, indications for clinical usage are highlighted (Rapkin and Akopians 2012).

In the past 20 years of private practice, countless women suffering with PMS and menopausal tension, irritability and depressed mood have improved multiple symptoms with single or blended essential oils of clary sage, rose, geranium, neroli and ylang-ylang as inhalations and/or lower abdominal massages. Initial inhalations reduce the irritability, and longer-lasting effects come with three months of twice-daily treatments beginning on day 14, the start of menstrual flow. Women accustomed to clear directions for the use of prescribed medications and treatments appreciate simple guidelines such as the following examples:

- Inhale for 2–5 minutes at least twice a day.

- Apply blended lotion to lower abdomen and around wrists twice a day during the last two weeks of your cycle.

- Add 4–6 drops to milk, then pour into your bath as you enter; bathe for a minimum of 20 minutes.

- Apply at least one teaspoon (5 ml) of blended lotion directly to the area of discomfort and massage for 1–2 minutes as often as needed.

- For panic or nausea, inhale 2–10 minutes as needed until symptoms improve.

In my clinical experience, women only need initial instructions; they can then determine the amounts and frequency that work best for them. With clear nursing and midwifery guidelines to initiate treatment, women view the therapy in a more positive manner as a legitimate healing modality.

# CHAPTER 6

# Aromatherapy for Menstrual Discomforts

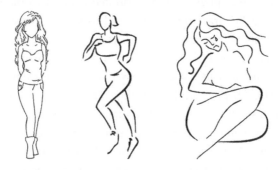

Young women starting from menarche, and sometimes for decades after, suffer from various menstrual discomforts ranging from mild monthly menstrual cramps to raging PMS. As a young teenage girl starts her period, our messages to her about her body will stay with her for a lifetime. The "blessing" of a female body (as opposed to the "curse") highlights the specialness of being a female and promotes a healthier body image.

The discomforts are real, occurring monthly for many, and can be completely incapacitating, leading to school and work absences as well as negatively affecting relationships and quality of life. Among adolescent girls, studies report a 50–90% incidence of primary dysmenorrhea (Sharma *et al.* 2008), lower abdominal pain occurring prior to the onset of menses without identifiable structural or hormonal pathology. Overall, dysmenorrhea, one of the most common gynecologic conditions, affects more than half of all women.

A survey of US women aged 18–44 indicated that 67% used at least one complementary alternative medicine (CAM) therapy, with aromatherapy highlighted as the therapy most often used for dysmenorrhea, i.e. menstrual pain and discomfort (Johnson *et al.* 2016). The chemical complexity of essential oils provides various therapeutic properties such as analgesic, antispasmodic, circulatory stimulant and sedative properties, thus altering pain perception and pathways (Marzouk *et al.* 2013). Women enjoy scents they experience as pleasant and relaxing, which enhance their sense of well-being. Aromatherapy eases unpleasant sensations while providing gentle physical and emotional comfort to the young teen, easing her transition from a girl to young woman while educating her on the options for self-care.

Lighter essential oils such as lemon, lavender, mandarin and bergamot inhaled in a room diffuser or bath are calming and uplifting for a happier adolescent. Teens enjoy choosing their own oils from a small collection and self-treating as needed. Diffusing or spritzing common, personal or study areas prior to a teen's return home from school or practice alters the angst of long, sometimes difficult days. Personal space can be improved with a collection of self-made blends based on their scent preferences. Diffusers for focus or study and uplifting or calming blends can be available as they deem necessary and signal underlying emotional states to parents. Teens are dealing with so many personal issues, often intensified by family dynamics, which I have found to be helped with aromatherapy.

The physical and emotional discomforts of the monthly cycle can be frightening, unpredictable and debilitating for the adolescent. The pleasant variety of scents offers individual choice and ability to have control to improve the unpleasant situation and enhance personal space. Inhalation of citrus oils (mandarin, bergamot, lemon) or lavender singly or in blends acts quickly to offset sudden, strong emotions and decrease perception of pain. Massage to the lower abdomen with analgesic and antispasmodic oils in lotion acts quickly to dull the pain and cramping. These methods have been successful for decades in my practice with sedentary young woman as well as competitive athletes.

## Menstrual cycle/dysmenorrhea list of clinically evidence-based essential oils

- Cinnamon (*Cinnamomum zeylancium*)

- Clary sage (*Salvia sclarea*)

- Clove (*Syzygium aromaticum*)

- Geranium (*Pelargonium graveolens*)

- Lavender (*Lavandula angustifolia*)

- Rose (*Rosa damascena*)

- Sweet marjoram (*Origanum marjoram*)

## Essential oils for menstrual cycle discomfort
### Cinnamon (Cinnamomum zeylancium)
Warm, familiar culinary spice oil.

**Safety:** Skin sensitivity occurrences with cinnamon (especially bark) indicate caution and low percentages (0.5–1%) when using this oil.

**Method of application:** Massage.

**Research:** In all of the studies, cinnamon has been added to a blend for abdominal massage that has been shown to ease discomfort more than massage alone and decrease the need for oral analgesics.

* Hur, M.H., Lee, M.S., Seong, K.Y. and Lee, M.K. (2012) "Aromatherapy massage on the abdomen for alleviating menstrual pain in high school girls: A preliminary controlled clinical study." *Evidence-Based Complementary and Alternative Medicine*, Epub 2012:187163.

* Marzouk, T.M., El-Nemer, A.M. and Baraka, H.N. (2013) "The effect of aromatherapy abdominal massage on alleviating menstrual pain in nursing students: A prospective randomized cross-over study." *Evidence-Based Complementary and Alternative Medicine*, Epub 2013:742421.

## Clary sage (Salvia sclarea)

Potent musky sage-like scent.

**Safety:** Euphoric; avoid using heavy machinery after use. Phytoestrogenic properties; therefore avoid during pregnancy or with history of reproductive cancer. If endometriosis or estrogen dominance is an issue, be cautious with clary sage.

**Method of application:** Massage.

**Research:** All of the studies with clary sage were blends of 3–6 essential oils diluted for an abdominal massage and shown to be more effective at easing dysmenorrhea than carrier oil alone, or acetaminophen (as compared by Hur *et al.* 2012): Han *et al.* (2006) (clary sage, rose and lavender), Hur *et al.* (2012) (clary sage, marjoram, cinnamon, ginger and geranium) and Ou *et al.* (2012) (clary sage, lavender and marjoram).

* Han, S.H., Hur, M.H., Buckle, J., Choi, J. and Lee, M.S. (2006) "Effect of aromatherapy on symptoms of dysmenorrhea in college students; a randomized placebo controlled trial." *Journal of Alternative and Complementary Medicine 12*, 6, 535–541.

* Hur, M.H., Lee, M.S., Seong, K.Y. and Lee, M.K. (2012) "Aromatherapy massage on the abdomen for alleviating

menstrual pain in high school girls: A preliminary controlled clinical study." *Evidence-Based Complementary and Alternative Medicine*, Epub 2012:187163.

* Ou, M.C., Hsu, T.F., Lai, A.C., Lin, Y.T. and Lin, C.C. (2012) "Pain relief assessment by aromatic essential oil massage on outpatients with primary dysmenorrhea: A randomized, double-blind clinical trial." *Journal of Obstetrics and Gynaecology Research 38*, 5, 817–822.

## Clove (Syzygium aromaticum)

Sweet, familiar culinary spice scent.

**Therapeutic properties:** An analgesic, anesthetic spice oil, historically used for toothache and teething pain, isolating eugenol in a topical anesthetic gel. Clove has not been commonly used in nursing aromatherapy blends.

**Method of application:** Massage.

**Research:** In Marzouk *et al.* (2013) clove in a massage blend of four oils decreased pain and menstrual bleeding in the first three days of the menses significantly greater than massage alone. The local anesthetic and increased circulation properties of clove were discussed as potential therapeutic actions.

* Marzouk, T.M., El-Nemer, A.M. and Baraka, H.N. (2013) "The effect of aromatherapy abdominal massage on alleviating menstrual pain in nursing students: A prospective randomized cross-over study." *Evidence-Based Complementary and Alternative Medicine*, Epub 2013:742421.

## Geranium (Pelargonium graveolens)

Strong floral scent.

**Therapeutic properties:** Uplifting and physically and emotionally balancing during hormonal upheaval. Eases fluid retention.

**Method of application:** Massage.

**Research:** The study blend included geranium (clary sage, marjoram, cinnamon, ginger and geranium) in an abdominal massage, effective in reducing menstrual pain significantly more than acetaminophen oral analgesic.

* Hur, M.H., Lee, M.S., Seong, K.Y. and Lee, M.K. (2012) "Aromatherapy massage on the abdomen for alleviating menstrual pain in high school girls: A preliminary controlled clinical study." *Evidence-Based Complementary and Alternative Medicine,* Epub 2012:187163.

## Lavender (Lavandula angustifolia)

Familiar, clean, herbaceous, floral.

**Therapeutic properties:** Multiple physical and emotional healing and balancing effects.

**Method of application:** Inhalation, massage.

**Research:** In Nikjou *et al.*'s (2016) study of 200 young women aged 19–29, inhalations of lavender for 30 minutes a day, on days 1–3 of the menstrual cycle for two consecutive cycles, was shown to significantly improve pain levels more than the control group; none used additional analgesics. Apay *et al.* (2012) and Bakhtshirin *et al.* (2015) also found lavender abdominal massage to relieve dysmenorrhea significantly more than massage alone. Raisi Dehkordi *et al.* (2014) observed that diluted lavender rubbed on to the hands and inhaled for five minutes every six hours, beginning one hour after experiencing dysmenorrhea for the first three days of menstruation, was statistically more effective at relieving primary dysmenorrhea than the control group, but did not significantly decrease menstrual flow. In a meta-analysis of six RCTs (n = 362) Sut and Kahyaoglu-Sut (2017) found that aromatherapy massage with lavender was superior to placebo at relieving pain in primary dysmenorrhea and that lavender alone in massage was more effective than massage with other oils blended with lavender. Other studies (Han *et al.* 2006; Ou *et al.* 2012) found that lavender blended with other oils in abdominal massage was, in all cases, more effective at relieving pain than placebo, and Marzouk *et al.* (2013) noted decreased menstrual bleeding in addition to decreased pain in the aromatherapy massage group.

* Apay, S.E., Arslan, S., Akpinar, R.B. and Celebioglu, A. (2012) "Effect of aromatherapy massage on dysmenorrhea in Turkish students." *Pain Management Nursing 13*, 4, 236–240.

* Bakhtshirin, F., Abedi, S., YusefiZoj, P. and Razmjooee, D. (2015) "The effect of aromatherapy massage with lavender oil on severity of primary dysmenorrhea in Arsanjan students." *Iranian Journal of Nursing and Midwifery Research 20*, 1, 156–160.

* Han, S.H., Hur, M.H., Buckle, J., Choi, J. and Lee, M.S. (2006) "Effect of aromatherapy on symptoms of dysmenorrhea in college students; a randomized placebo controlled trial." *Journal of Alternative and Complementary Medicine 12*, 6, 535–541.

* Marzouk, T.M.F., El-Nemer, A.M.R. and Baraka, H.N. (2013) "The effect of aromatherapy abdominal massage on alleviating menstrual pain in nursing students: A prospective randomized cross-over study." *Evidence-Based Complementary and Alternative Medicine*, Epub 2013:742421.

* Nikjou, R., Kazemzadeh, R., Rostamnegad, M., Moshfegi, S., Karimollahi, M. and Salehi, H. (2016) "The effect of lavender aromatherapy on the pain severity of primary dysmenorrhea: A triple-blind randomized clinical trial."*Annals of Medical and Health Sciences Research 6*, 4, 211–215.

* Ou, M.C., Hsu, T.F., Lai, A.C., Lin, Y.T. and Lin, C.C. (2012) "Pain relief assessment by aromatic essential oil massage on outpatients with primary dysmenorrhea: A randomized, double-blind clinical trial." *Journal of Obstetrics and Gynaecology Research 38*, 5, 817–822.

* Raisi Dehkordi, Z., Hosseini Baharanchi, F.S. and Bekhradi, R. (2014) "Effect of lavender inhalation on the symptoms of primary dysmenorrhea and the amount of menstrual bleeding: A randomized clinical trial." *Complementary Therapies in Medicine 22*, 2, 212–219.

* Sut, N. and Kahyaoglu-Sut, H. (2017) "Effect of aromatherapy massage on pain in primary dysmenorrhea: A meta-analysis." *Complementary Therapies in Clinical Practice 27*, 5–10.

## Rose (Rosa damascena)

Strong, sweet, floral.

**Therapeutic properties:** Known as the "queen of flowers," with affinity for the female reproductive system from menarche to menopause; often associated with older women through childhood memories.

**Method of application:** Inhalation, massage.

**Research:** In a study by Sadeghi Aval Shahr *et al.* (2015), self-massage with and without rose oil was completed on the first day of menstruation for two consecutive cycles, with statistically significant improvement noted in the rose oil group after the second cycle, greater than massage without rose oil or with no treatment at all. Uysal *et al.* (2016) found that vaporized rose oil combined with medication was more effective pain relief than the same medication alone. Marzouk *et al.* (2013) (cinnamon, clove, rose and lavender) and Han *et al.* (2006) (rose, lavender and clary sage) combined rose otto in abdominal massage blends with other essential oils, all showing significant reduction of pain, greater than abdominal massage without essential oils.

* Han, S.H., Hur, M.H., Buckle, J., Choi, J. and Lee, M.S. (2006) "Effect of aromatherapy on symptoms of dysmenorrhea in college students; a randomized placebo controlled trial." *Journal of Alternative and Complementary Medicine 12,* 6, 535–541.

* Marzouk, T.M.F., El-Nemer, A.M.R. and Baraka, H.N. (2013) "The effect of aromatherapy abdominal massage on alleviating menstrual pain in nursing students: A prospective randomized cross-over study." *Evidence-Based Complementary and Alternative Medicine,* Epub 2013:742421.

* Sadeghi Aval Shahr, H., Saadat, M., Kheirkhah, M. and Saadat, E. (2015) "The effect of self-aromatherapy massage of the abdomen on the primary dysmenorrhea." *Journal of Obstetrics and Gynaecology 35,* 4, 382–385.

* Uysal, M., Doğru, H.Y., Sapmaz, E., Tas, U. *et al.* (2016) "Investigating the effect of rose essential oil in patients with primary dysmenorrhea." *Complementary Therapies in Clinical Practice 24,* 45–49.

## Sweet marjoram (Oreganum marjoram)
Sweet, woody, herbal.

**Therapeutic properties:** Relaxing and clinically supportive in pain blends for minor muscular injuries, pains and menstrual discomforts.

**Method of application:** Massage.

**Research:** In studies, in an abdominal massage blend, sweet marjoram has been shown to be effective at reducing pain and need for acetaminophen oral analgesics.

* Hur, M.H., Lee, M.S., Seong, K.Y. and Lee, M.K. (2012) "Aromatherapy massage on the abdomen for alleviating menstrual pain in high school girls: A preliminary controlled clinical study." *Evidence-Based Complementary and Alternative Medicine*, Epub 2012:187163.

* Ou, M.C., Hsu, T.F., Lai, A.C., Lin, Y.T. and Lin, C.C. (2012) "Pain relief assessment by aromatic essential oil massage on outpatients with primary dysmenorrhea: A randomized, double-blind clinical trial." *Journal of Obstetrics and Gynaecology Research 38*, 5, 817–822.

## Menstrual blends
### Heavy menstrual flow
Lemon 2 drops, lavender 2 drops, cypress 1 drop in 5 ml lotion.

### Menstrual cramps
Lavender 2 drops, clary sage 1 drop, rose 1 drop in 5 ml lotion (Han *et al.* 2006 blend).

Lavender 2 drops, Roman chamomile 1 drop, sweet marjoram 1 drop in 5 ml lotion.

### Fluid retention
Geranium 2 drops, mandarin 2 drops in 5 ml lotion.

### Sadness, mild depression
Lavender 3 drops, rose 1 drop in 10 ml jojoba oil. Put 4–6 drops on a cotton pad and inhale throughout the day for 2–5 minutes at a time.

Lavender 1 drop, lemon 1 drop in 5 ml jojoba oil. Put 4–6 drops on a cotton pad and inhale throughout the day.

Mandarin 1 drop, bergamot 1 drop, lemon 1 drop. Add 6–12 drops of blend to 1 oz glass bottle, add distilled water, shake and spray around yourself 2–4 times/day. Inhale and enjoy.

Young women respond exceptionally well to aromatherapy for menstrual issues and prefer this method to oral analgesics. The combination of self-care, essential oil choice, strength of blend and pleasant scents enhances the experience and quality of life. In my private practice, consistent use of select individual oils and/or blends in varied methods has shown significant improvement of symptoms within weeks or months.

## Quick reference table: menstrual discomforts

| Condition | Essential oils (blends of 1–3) | Methods |
|---|---|---|
| Abdominal heaviness, fluid retention | Geranium, lavender, sweet marjoram | Lower abdominal massage prior to menses |
| Menstrual cramps | Lavender, sweet marjoram, clary sage, cinnamon, clove | Lower abdominal massage as needed |
| Heavy menstrual flow | Lavender, clove | Inhalation on cotton pad and lower abdominal massage days 1–3 of period |
| Sadness, mild depression | Rose, lavender, clary sage, geranium, yuzu | Inhalation on cotton pad, diffuser, spritzer |

# CHAPTER 7

# Aromatherapy for Premenstrual Syndrome (PMS)

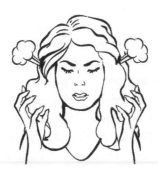

A week to ten days prior to the onset of their period, the *luteal phase* of the cycle, the majority of women of reproductive age are prone to experiencing a cluster of mild to severe physical and emotional symptoms known as premenstrual syndrome or PMS. The shifting progesterone and estrogen levels, imbalanced in many women, are the culprit for intense feelings of irritability, tension, depression, heightened stress, often described as "I feel like I'm jumping out of my skin" or, at its worst, "I'm going to rip your face off": pure misery for the woman as well as those in her personal or professional paths. Being physically uncomfortable with fluid retention, breast tenderness, weight gain, bloating, gastrointestinal changes and abdominal pain makes women feel miserable on a monthly basis for years. PMS in modern times has an incidence of 40–80% of women worldwide and is documented as far back as Hippocrates (520–460 BC).

The Association of Women's Health, Obstetric and Neonatal Nurses (AWHONN) label this collection of symptoms "cyclic perimenstrual pain and discomfort" (CPPD), reflecting the dynamic nature of symptoms (Collins Sharp *et al.* 2002). Multiple studies estimate a global incidence of 80–97% of women experiencing at least one symptom at some point in their reproductive life (Halbreich 2003; Ju *et al.* 2014; Milewicz and Jedrzejuk 2006; Wittchen *et al.* 2002). Multiple days lost from work and school and, at its extreme, serious psychological dysfunction can be the reality for many women.

The effect of PMS on the endocrine, psychological and nervous systems from increases in cortisol, decreases in serotonin and estrogen/progesterone imbalance are well documented. Aromatherapy research studies measuring pre- and post-levels of stress hormones, and positively correlating them with self-reported changes in mood states, provide a potential mechanism of action for aromatherapy on a physiological level and offer a valid tool for easing the many discomforts of PMS. As most women (and many men) are aware, PMS is miserable and at times can be frightening. As a result of the high incidence of occurrence and women's concerns about risk factors with pharmaceuticals, many self-treat with CAM, and women are particularly fond of aromatherapy as a self-care modality.

## PMS list of clinically evidence-based essential oils

- Lavender (*Lavandula angustifolia*)

- Yuzu (*Citrus junos*)

### Lavender (*Lavandula angustifolia*)
Familiar soft, herbaceous, floral scent.

**Therapeutic properties:** The calming and sedative properties of lavender soothe the angst, tension and irritability of PMS. Studies indicate that inhalations improve self-reported scores for PMS stress, anxiety and depression.

**Method of application:** Inhalation.

**Research:** Uzuncakmak and Alkaya (2017) showed that lavender steam inhalations once daily, starting ten days before the start of menstruation until menstrual flow begins, for three consecutive cycles resulted in significant improvements in PMS anxiety, depressive affect and thoughts, pain and bloating. Matsumoto *et al.* (2013) measured effects on the parasympathetic nervous system of ten-minute lavender inhalations by women experiencing PMS in the late luteal phase. Significant rapid improvements were noted in heart rate variability (HRV), showing parasympathetic response as well as improvement in self-reported symptoms of depression, dejection and confusion as measured by the Profile of Mood States (POMS; Yokoyama and Araki 1994). Matsumoto *et al.* (2017) compared parasympathetic activity and self-reported POMS with ten-minute inhalations of yuzu and lavender, which both indicated significant reduction in heart rate, tension, anxiety, anger, hostility and fatigue. The yuzu and lavender inhalations had very similar responses so could both be used for the emotional symptoms of PMS.

★ Matsumoto, T., Asakura, H. and Hayashi, T. (2013) "Does lavender aromatherapy alleviate premenstrual emotional symptoms? A randomized crossover trial." *Biopsychosocial Medicine* 7, 1, 12.

★ Matsumoto, T., Kimura, T. and Hayashi, T. (2017) "Does Japanese citrus fruit yuzu (Citrus junos Sieb. ex Tanaka) fragrance have lavender-like therapeutic effects that alleviate premenstrual emotional symptoms? A single-blind randomized crossover study." *Journal of Alternative and Complementary Medicine* 23, 6, 461–470.

* Uzuncakmak, T. and Alkaya, S.A. (2017) "Effect of aromatherapy on coping with premenstrual syndrome: A randomized controlled trial." *Complementary Therapies in Medicine 36*, 63–67.

* Yokoyama, K. and Araki, S. (1994) *A Manual of the Japanese Translation of POMS.* Tokyo: Kaneko Shobo.

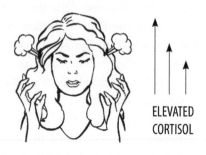

ELEVATED
CORTISOL

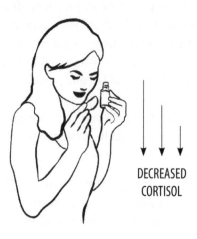

DECREASED
CORTISOL

## Yuzu (Citrus junos)

Fresh, soft, floral.

**Therapeutic properties:** Uplifting welcome option for anxiety, depression and overall well-being.

**Method of application:** Inhalation.

**Research:** Matsumoto *et al.* (2017) studied women with PMS who completed ten-minute inhalations of yuzu during the luteal phase; findings were comparable to the relaxing effects of lavender, with parasympathetic responses of decreased heart rate and HRV, as well as POMS self-reported improvement of tension, anxiety, anger, hostility and fatigue.

★ Matsumoto, T., Kimura, T. and Hayashi, T. (2017) "Does Japanese citrus fruit yuzu (Citrus junos Sieb. ex Tanaka) fragrance have lavender-like therapeutic effects that alleviate premenstrual emotional symptoms? A single-blind randomized crossover study." *Journal of Alternative and Complementary Medicine 23*, 6, 461–470.

The immediate reduction of the intense emotional symptoms of PMS supports the use of aromatherapy as a "go to" first response with the emergence of monthly symptoms. In my clinical practice, I repeatedly witness this response with multiple relaxing essential oils such as rose, lavender, ylang-ylang, clary sage, geranium, frankincense and neroli, which all have clinical evidence of reducing stress and anxiety. The ongoing evidence of inhalation with calming essential oils, reducing levels of CgA, cortisol and adrenaline, and improving mood states associated with PMS, supports aromatherapy as a self-care treatment option.

# Quick reference table: menstrual discomforts and premenstrual syndrome

| Condition | Essential oils (blends of 1–3) | Methods |
|---|---|---|
| Anger, tension, irritability | Lavender, yuzu, clary sage, geranium, rose | Inhalation on cotton pad; dilute in lotion, dab under nose and rub around wrists and ankles |
| Anxiety | Lavender, rose, geranium, yuzu, sweet marjoram, clary sage | Inhalation on cotton pad, massage, spritzer |
| Abdominal heaviness, fluid retention | Geranium, lavender, sweet marjoram | Lower abdominal massage prior to menses |
| Menstrual cramps | Lavender, sweet marjoram, clary sage, cinnamon, clove | Lower abdominal massage as needed |
| Heavy menstrual flow | Lavender, clove | Inhalation on cotton pad and lower abdominal massage days 1–3 of period |
| Sadness, mild depression | Rose, lavender, clary sage, geranium, yuzu | Inhalation on cotton pad, diffuser, spritzer |

# CHAPTER 8

# Aromatherapy for Menopause

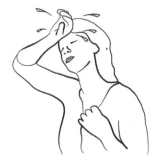

Menopause is defined as the end of the reproductive years with the absence of menses for one continuous year. The average age for menopause is 51, with some women experiencing physical and emotional symptoms for up to ten years prior to the complete cessation of menstrual flow, known as the "perimenopause period." The rapidly declining ovarian production of estrogen shifts the delicate hormonal balance, with marginal amounts being produced from the adrenal glands. Classic physical menopausal symptoms include vasomotor hot flashes and night sweats leading to loss of sleep and constant sensations of rising heat, and vaginal changes with dryness, decreased elasticity and atrophy, leading to painful intercourse. There are accompanying emotional symptoms of depression and confusion, and increased risk factors for cardiovascular events and osteoporosis. Women also sadly notice hair and skin changes that highlight the often-unwelcome aging process. The question of how best to treat any or all of these symptoms is quite a challenge.

## Neurotransmitters, hormones and women's health aromatherapy

Multiple aromatherapy studies (Chen *et al.* 2017; Hosseini *et al.* 2016; Hur *et al.* 2012; Lee *et al.* 2014; Watanabe *et al.* 2015) have shown decreases in salivary cortisol (stress hormone), and increases in serotonin 5HT ("antidepressant neurotransmitter") and estrogen levels with inhalation and massage aromatherapy treatments.

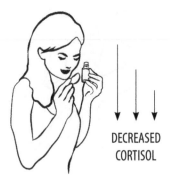

DECREASED CORTISOL

Researchers are extending their inquiries beyond self-reported pre- and post-aromatherapy treatment scores to measure physiologic salivary and serum levels. In these studies, symptoms resulting from elevated cortisol and serotonin deficiency, and severity of PMS and menopausal symptoms were all improved with simple aromatherapy inhalations and massage treatments. The treatment duration ranged from single treatments to twice weekly for 12 weeks, and there were longer-term improvements. These results offer short- and long-term therapeutic options with minimal risks and lasting effects.

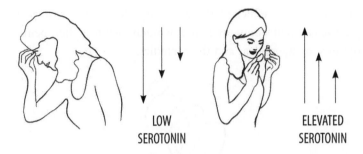

LOW
SEROTONIN

ELEVATED
SEROTONIN

Historically, menopausal women were prescribed HRT: the same dosage of the same medications, premarin and progestin, for all women—rather a one-size-fits-all. In 2002, this all changed when the Women's Health Initiative (WHI) multicenter study evaluating the major risks and benefits of the hormone preparation that had been prescribed in the US for decades was prematurely discontinued. The findings indicated increased risks of coronary heart disease (CHD), stroke, pulmonary embolism and breast cancer with HRT. The Heart Estrogen Replacement Study (HERS) also indicated an increased CHD incidence in the first year (Roussow *et al.* 2002). Celebrex and Vioxx, widely prescribed medications for chronic pain, were revealed to increase serious heart disease and stroke risk, and were taken off the market (Sibbald 2004). Antidepressant prescription medications were also found to increase the risk of suicide in young adults, further raising overall fears of pharmaceuticals (Hammad 2006).

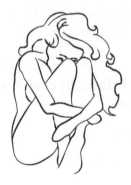

The cumulative effect of these findings led to mistrust with pharmaceutical companies and women seeking therapeutic options for themselves and their families.

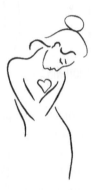

A survey of more than 10,000 women aged 59–64 indicated that 75% used self-prescribed CAM with nearly 40% consulting a CAM practitioner (Peng *et al.* 2014). Aromatherapy oils were more likely to be used for anxiety and hot flashes than other CAM modalities.

Fluctuating levels of estrogen, cortisol and serotonin are thought to be contributing factors in the physical and psychological symptoms of menopause. As will be demonstrated in the following evidence review, multiple aromatherapy studies have shown that select essential oils affect hormonal and neurotransmitter levels with noted improvements in menopausal symptoms. Inhalation and aromatherapy massage were the methods utilized for 5–30 minutes duration, once or twice daily, for five days over the course of eight weeks, all with positive outcomes.

## Menopause list of clinically evidence-based essential oils

- Bergamot (*Citrus bergamia*)
- Clary sage (*Salvia sclarea*)

- Cypress (*Cupressus sempervirens*)

- Geranium (*Pelargonium graveolens*)

- Jasmine (*Jasminum grandiflorum or Jasminum sambac*)

- Lavender (*Lavandula angustifolia*)

- Mandarin (*Citrus reticulata*)

- Neroli (*Citrus aurantium var. amara*)

- Peppermint (*Mentha piperita*)

- Roman chamomile (*Anthemis nobilis*)

- Rosemary (*Rosmarinus officinalis*)

- Rose (*Rosa damascena*)

- Ylang-ylang (*Cananga odorata*)

- Yuzu (*Citrus junos*)

## Essential oils for menopause
### Bergamot (*Citrus bergania*)
Scent is woody, bitter citrus.

**Therapeutic properties:** Uplifting and calming for stress, depression and anxiety.

**Method of application:** Massage.

**Research:** Menopausal depressive symptoms on the Kupperman Index (KI) were improved after two massages one month apart for various oils including bergamot in Murakami *et al.*'s (2005) study.

- ★ Murakami, S., Shirota, T., Hayashi, S. and Ishizuka, B. (2005) "Aromatherapy for outpatients with menopausal symptoms in obstetrics and gynecology." *Journal of Alternative and Complementary Medicine 11*, 3, 491–494.

## Clary sage (Salvia sclarea)

Strong musky, sage-like herbal scent.

**Therapeutic properties:** Euphorically calming for stress, anxiety and hormonal angst.

**Safety:** Clary sage is profoundly relaxing and euphoric, and caution with operating heavy machinery is advised. Potentiates alcohol. Avoid during pregnancy or with history of reproductive cancers due to phytoestrogenic properties.

**Method of application:** Massage, inhalation.

**Research:** Lee *et al.* (2014) found that after inhalation cortisol levels were significantly decreased and 5HT/serotonin was significantly increased, demonstrating the antidepressant (5HT) and cortisol-reducing potential of clary sage in menopausal women. Seo and Park (2003) demonstrated that inhalation of two drops on a pad every four hours during the day for two weeks achieved significant reductions in the physical and psychological menopausal symptom scales, positively supporting use for stress in menopause. In Murakami *et al.*'s (2005) study, menopausal depressive symptoms on the Kupperman Index (KI) were improved after two massages one month apart for various oils, including clary sage.

* Lee, K.B., Cho, E. and Kang, Y.S. (2014) "Changes in 5-hydroxytryptamine and cortisol plasma levels in menopausal women after inhalation of clary sage oil." *Phytotherapy Research 28*, 11, 1599–1605.

* Murakami, S., Shirota, T., Hayashi, S. and Ishizuka, B. (2005) "Aromatherapy for outpatients with menopausal symptoms in obstetrics and gynecology." *Journal of Alternative and Complementary Medicine 11*, 3, 491–494.

* Seo, H.K. and Park, K.S. (2003) "A study on the effects of aroma inhalation method using Clarysage essential oil on stress in middle-aged women." *Korean Journal of Women Health Nursing 9*, 1, 70–79.

## Cypress *(Cupressus sempervirens)*

Evergreen with a fresh woody scent.

**Therapeutic properties:** Astringent properties ease perspiration, excess menstrual flow and fluid retention.

**Method of application:** Massage.

**Research:** In Lee (2002), a blend of geranium, Roman chamomile and cypress showed improvements of menopausal symptoms with two aromatherapy massages, one month apart.

* ★ Lee, S.H. (2002) "Effects of aromatherapy massage on depression, self-esteem, climacteric symptoms in the middle aged women." *Korean Journal of Women Health Nursing 8,* 2, 278–288.

## Geranium *(Pelargonium graveolens)*

Strong floral aroma.

**Therapeutic properties:** Appreciated by women for its emotional and physical balancing effects associated with menopause.

**Method of application:** Inhalation, massage.

**Research:** Shinohara *et al.* (2017) studied the effects of inhalation of various essential oils (clary sage, frankincense, geranium, lavender, jasmine absolute, neroli, rose, ylang-ylang, orange and Roman chamomile) on estrogen concentration. The results demonstrated an increase of salivary estrogen concentration, specifically with exposure to geranium and rose essential oils compared with the control odor. Aromatherapy massage with essential oil blends containing geranium in the other studies demonstrated improvement of physical and emotional menopausal symptoms. Clinically, we have also experienced geranium as an aid for fluid retention with aromatherapy massage.

★ Darsareh, F., Taavoni, S., Joolaee, S. and Haghani, H. (2012) "Effect of aromatherapy massage on menopausal symptoms: A randomized placebo-controlled clinical trial." *Menopause 19*, 9, 995–999.

★ Hur, M.H., Yang, Y.S. and Lee, M.S. (2008) "Aromatherapy massage affects menopausal symptoms in Korean climacteric women: A pilot-controlled clinical trial." *Evidence-Based Complementary and Alternative Medicine 5*, 3, 325–328.

★ Kim, S., Song, J.A., Kim, M.E. and Hur, M.H. (2016) "Effects of aromatherapy on menopausal symptoms, perceived stress and depression in middle-aged women: A systematic review." *Journal of Korean Academy of Nursing 46*, 5, 619–629.

★ Murakami, S., Shirota, T., Hayashi, S. and Ishizuka, B. (2005) "Aromatherapy for outpatients with menopausal symptoms in obstetrics and gynecology." *Journal of Alternative and Complementary Medicine 11*, 3, 491–494.

★ Shinohara, K., Doi, H., Kumagai, C., Sawano, E. and Tarumi, W. (2017) "Effects of essential oil exposure on salivary estrogen concentration in perimenopausal women." *Neuro Endocrinology Letters 37*, 8, 567–572.

★ Taavoni, S., Darsareh, F., Joolaee, S. and Haghani, H. (2013) "The effect of aromatherapy massage on the psychological symptoms of postmenopausal Iranian women." *Complementary Therapies in Medicine 21*, 3, 158–163.

## *Jasmine (Jasminum officinale)*

Sensual and strengthening exotic floral.

**Therapeutic properties:** Sensual and emotionally strengthening. Uplifting and supportive with depression. Therapeutic perfume enhances well-being.

**Method of application:** Massage, inhalation.

**Research:** Hur *et al.*'s (2008) study of a weekly massage with blended oils (jasmine, rose, geranium, lavender) for eight weeks showed improvements on the Kupperman Index (KI) for menopausal pain, depression and hot flashes. Clinically, women often report improved mood and increased psychological strength with 2–4% jasmine inhalations.

* Hur, M.H., Yang, Y.S. and Lee, M.S. (2008) "Aromatherapy massage affects menopausal symptoms in Korean climacteric women: A pilot-controlled clinical trial." *Evidence-Based Complementary and Alternative Medicine 5*, 3, 325–328.

* Kim, S., Song, J.A., Kim, M.E. and Hur, M.H. (2016) "Effects of aromatherapy on menopausal symptoms, perceived stress and depression in middle-aged women: A systematic review." *Journal of Korean Academy of Nursing 46*, 5, 619–629.

## *Lavender (Lavandula angutifolia)*
Soft, floral, herbal.

**Therapeutic properties:** The calming properties of lavender identified in the studies and in my practice are especially helpful to reduce the stress and changes of menopause.

**Method of application:** Inhalation, massage.

**Research:** Kazemzadeh *et al.* (2016) reported that twice-daily 20-minute lavender inhalations for 12 weeks decreased hot flashes in menopausal women by 50%. The other studies of essential oil massage blends included lavender, with significant improvements in physical and psychological menopausal symptoms. The intensity, frequency and duration of hot flashes and night sweats, tension and irritability are quickly improved with inhalation or with the cooling skin contact of a lavender spritzer.

* Darsareh, F., Taavoni, S., Joolaee, S. and Haghani, H. (2012) "Effect of aromatherapy massage on menopausal symptoms: A randomized placebo-controlled clinical trial." *Menopause 19*, 9, 995–999.

* Hur, M.H., Yang, Y.S. and Lee, M.S. (2008) "Aromatherapy massage affects menopausal symptoms in Korean climacteric women: A pilot-controlled clinical trial." *Evidence-Based Complementary and Alternative Medicine 5*, 3, 325–328.

* Kazemzadeh, R., Nikjou, R., Rostamnegad, M. and Nourouzi, H. (2016) "Effect of lavender aromatherapy on menopause hot flushing: a crossover randomized clinical trial." *Journal of the Chinese Medical Association 79*, 9, 489–492.

* Kim, S., Song, J.A., Kim, M.E. and Hur, M.H. (2016) "Effects of aromatherapy on menopausal symptoms, perceived stress and depression in middle-aged women: A systematic review." *Journal of Korean Academy of Nursing 46*, 5, 619–629.

* Murakami, S., Shirota, T., Hayashi, S. and Ishizuka, B. (2005) "Aromatherapy for outpatients with menopausal symptoms in obstetrics and gynecology." *Journal of Alternative and Complementary Medicine 11*, 3, 491–494.

* Taavoni, S., Darsareh, F., Joolaee, S. and Haghani, H. (2013) "The effect of aromatherapy massage on the psychological symptoms of postmenopausal Iranian women." *Complementary Therapies in Medicine 21*, 3, 158–163.

## Mandarin (Citrus reticulata)

Soft citrus scent.

**Therapeutic properties:** Gently uplifting emotionally and eases abdominal discomforts from bloating, fluid retention and constipation.

**Method of application:** Massage.

**Research:** In a 30-minute massage with blended oils (mandarin, lavender, ylang-ylang) three times a week for two weeks improved scores were noted for physical and psychological menopausal symptoms (Son and Kim 2013).

* Son, H.O. and Kim, H.N. (2013) "Effects of aroma back massage on the relief of middle-aged women's stress." *Journal of the Korean Society of Esthetics and Cosmeceutics 8*, 2, 111–123.

## Neroli (Citrus aurantium)

Strong, citrus, floral.

**Therapeutic properties:** Eases panic, stress and anxiety often associated with hormonal imbalances.

**Method of application:** Inhalation.

**Research:** Choi *et al.*'s (2014) study showed that inhalations of 1–5% neroli twice a day for five days increased libido and quality of life; decreased diastolic blood pressure and pulse were reported.

* Choi, S.Y., Kang, P., Lee, H.S. and Seol, G.H. (2014) "Effects of inhalation of essential oil of Citrus aurantium l var. amara on menopausal symptoms, stress, and estrogen in postmenopausal women: A randomized controlled trial." *Evidence-Based Complementary and Alternative Medicine*, Epub 2014:796518.

* Murakami, S., Shirota, T., Hayashi, S. and Ishizuka, B. (2005) "Aromatherapy for outpatients with menopausal symptoms in obstetrics and gynecology." *Journal of Alternative and Complementary Medicine 11*, 3, 491–494.

## Peppermint (Mentha piperita)

Fresh culinary mint, familiar.

**Therapeutic properties:** A stimulating oil, refreshing as a popular and very effective inhalation for medical/surgical and migraine nausea.

**Method of application:** Massage.

**Research:** Menopausal depressive symptoms on the Kupperman Index (KI) were improved after two massages one month apart for various oils including peppermint in Murakami *et al.*'s (2005) study. In massage blends stress, pain and depression associated with menopause were improved.

★ Murakami, S., Shirota, T., Hayashi, S. and Ishizuka, B. (2005) "Aromatherapy for outpatients with menopausal symptoms in obstetrics and gynecology." *Journal of Alternative and Complementary Medicine 11*, 3, 491–494.

## Roman chamomile (Anthemis nobilis)

Herbal, grassy scent.

**Therapeutic properties:** A calming analgesic helpful for sleep, pain and abdominal and muscular cramping. Useful for a wide range of women's health issues.

**Method of application:** Massage.

**Research:** Lee (2002) noted improvements of menopausal symptoms with two aromatherapy massages, one month apart, using a blend of Roman chamomile, geranium and cypress.

★ Lee, S.H. (2002) "Effects of aromatherapy massage on depression, self-esteem, climacteric symptoms in the middle aged women." *Korean Journal of Women Health Nursing 8*, 2, 278–288.

★ Murakami, S., Shirota, T., Hayashi, S. and Ishizuka, B. (2005) "Aromatherapy for outpatients with menopausal symptoms in obstetrics and gynecology." *Journal of Alternative and Complementary Medicine 11*, 3, 491–494.

## Rosemary (Rosmarinus officinalis)

Refreshing camphor scent.

**Therapeutic properties:** "Rosemary for remembrance" was historically used for study and memory. Familiar in Mediterranean cuisine. Clinically, rosemary is a stimulating oil, enhancing focus and alertness as an inhalation and analgesic in pain blends.

**Method of application:** Massage.

**Research:** Studies by Darsareh *et al.* (2012) and Taavoni *et al.* (2013) measured psychological symptoms (irritability, exhaustion, anxiety and depressed mood, exhaustion) of menopausal women (age 45–60) with 3% massage blend (lavender, geranium, rose and rosemary) 30 minutes two times a week for four weeks. All symptoms significantly improved more in the aromatherapy group than massage alone, possibly due to expert selection of essential oils.

★ Darsareh, F., Taavoni, S., Joolaee, S. and Haghani, H. (2012) "Effect of aromatherapy massage on menopausal symptoms: A randomized placebo-controlled clinical trial." *Menopause 19*, 9, 995–999.

★ Taavoni, S., Darsareh, F., Joolaee, S. and Haghani, H. (2013) "The effect of aromatherapy massage on the psychological symptoms of postmenopausal Iranian women." *Complementary Therapies in Medicine 21*, 3, 158–163.

## Rose (Rosa damascena)

Strong, sweet, floral.

**Therapeutic properties:** Balancing female reproductive system during times of hormonal imbalance. Emotionally supportive with grief, depression and calming anxiety.

**Method of application:** Inhalation, massage.

**Research:** Shinohara *et al.* (2017) studied the effects of inhalation of various essential oils (clary sage, frankincense, geranium, lavender, jasmine absolute, neroli, rose, ylang-ylang, orange and Roman chamomile) on estrogen concentration. The results demonstrated an increase of salivary estrogen concentration specifically with exposure to geranium and rose essential oils compared with the control odor. Calming anxiety and irritability, improving depression and altering salivary estrogen levels were identified in the following studies through inhalation and massage.

* ★ Darsareh, F., Taavoni, S., Joolaee, S. and Haghani, H. (2012) "Effect of aromatherapy massage on menopausal symptoms: A randomized placebo-controlled clinical trial." *Menopause 19*, 9, 995–999.

* ★ Hur, M.H., Yang, Y.S. and Lee, M.S. (2008) "Aromatherapy massage affects menopausal symptoms in Korean climacteric women: A pilot-controlled clinical trial." *Evidence-Based Complementary and Alternative Medicine 5*, 3, 325–328.

* ★ Kim, S., Song, J.A., Kim, M.E. and Hur, M.H. (2016) "Effects of aromatherapy on menopausal symptoms, perceived stress and depression in middle-aged women: A systematic review." *Journal of Korean Academy of Nursing 46*, 5, 619–629.

* ★ Murakami, S., Shirota, T., Hayashi, S. and Ishizuka, B. (2005) "Aromatherapy for outpatients with menopausal symptoms

in obstetrics and gynecology." *Journal of Alternative and Complementary Medicine 11*, 3, 491–494.

★ Shinohara, K., Doi, H., Kumagai, C., Sawano, E. and Tarumi, W. (2017) "Effects of essential oil exposure on salivary estrogen concentration in perimenopausal women." *Neuro Endocrinology Letters 37*, 8, 567–572.

★ Taavoni, S., Darsareh, F., Joolaee, S. and Haghani, H. (2013) "The effect of aromatherapy massage on the psychological symptoms of postmenopausal Iranian women." *Complementary Therapies in Medicine 21*, 3, 158–163.

## Ylang-ylang *(Cananga odorata)*

Exotic, strong, floral scent.

**Therapeutic properties:** Eases anger, irritability and stress. Balancing with menopausal tachycardia and hypertension.

**Safety:** May cause headaches, best at 1–2%.

**Method of application:** Massage.

**Research:** Studied in a massage blend, it was shown to reduce stress and improve depression. Relaxing tension, anger, irritability, depression and stress is the strength of ylang-ylang in any women's health blend.

★ Kim, S., Song, J.A., Kim, M.E. and Hur, M.H. (2016) "Effects of aromatherapy on menopausal symptoms, perceived stress and depression in middle-aged women: A systematic review." *Journal of Korean Academy of Nursing 46*, 5, 619–629.

★ Murakami, S., Shirota, T., Hayashi, S. and Ishizuka, B. (2005) "Aromatherapy for outpatients with menopausal symptoms in obstetrics and gynecology." *Journal of Alternative and Complementary Medicine 11*, 3, 491–494.

## Yuzu (Citrus junos)

Soft, floral, citrus scent.

**Therapeutic properties:** Cheerful and uplifting with depression. Calming for anxiety and stress.

**Method of application:** Massage.

**Research:** Menopausal depressive symptoms on the Kupperman Index (KI) were improved after two massages one month apart for various oils including yuzu in Murakami *et al.*'s (2005) study.

★ Murakami, S., Shirota, T., Hayashi, S. and Ishizuka, B. (2005) "Aromatherapy for outpatients with menopausal symptoms in obstetrics and gynecology." *Journal of Alternative and Complementary Medicine 11*, 3, 491–494.

Aromatherapy for menopause encompasses the most luxurious essential oils with several options for the varied physical and emotional aspects of this rather long stage in a woman's life. Varying the oils every three weeks offers variety and greater effectiveness as hormone levels change. My personal and professional experience has demonstrated that scent preference and effectiveness can change from peri- to post-menopause, so continue to explore the options.

Enjoy the healing gift of aromatherapy to enhance your patients' lives as well your own and your loved ones'!

Aromatic blessings, Pam

# Quick reference table: menopause

| Condition | Essential oils (blends of 1–3) | Methods |
|---|---|---|
| Anxiety | Rose, lavender, geranium, neroli, ylang-ylang, yuzu, clary sage, mandarin, Roman chamomile | Inhalation on cotton pad or personal inhaler, diffuser, bath, massage, spritzer |
| Depression | Lavender, rose, jasmine, geranium, bergamot, mandarin, neroli, peppermint | Inhalation on cotton pad or personal inhaler, diffuser, spritzer, massage |
| Night sweats | Lavender, lemon, peppermint, cypress | Bath before bed, spritzer for cooling |
| Hot flashes | Clary sage, geranium, rose, lavender, peppermint, lemon, cypress | Inhalation on cotton pad for calming, spritzers for skin cooling |
| Irritability | Ylang-ylang, neroli, geranium, lavender, clary sage | Inhalation on cotton pad, shoulder or hand massage |
| Libido/sex drive | Jasmine, rose, lavender, ylang-ylang | Inhalation on cotton pad, couples' massages, room or sheet spritzer |
| Skin changes | Rose, lavender | Dilute 4% in lotion, apply to arms and legs |
| Grief | Rose, lavender | Inhalation on cotton pad, massage, bath |
| Heart palpitations/ tachycardia | Ylang-ylang, lavender | Inhalation on cotton pad, diffuser; always have evaluated by medical doctor |
| Difficulty concentrating/ focus | Rosemary, peppermint | Inhalation on cotton pad, diffuser, spritzer |
| Mood changes | Geranium, clary sage, rose, ylang-ylang | Inhalation on cotton pad, skin application shoulders, chest, wrists |

# Appendix

## Sample Clinical Aromatherapy Policy

### Policy statement

Aromatherapy is the art of using essential oils to help restore balance to the body. It is a complementary therapy, which aims to treat the whole person on a mental, physical and emotional level in order to promote health and well-being.

Essential oils are steam-distilled, expressed or extracted from various parts of aromatic plants.

### Educational requirements

Nurses or midwives as practitioners of complementary therapies must adhere to safe practice appropriate to their usual scope of practice, hospital policy and state board, in addition to those guidelines specific to the individual complementary therapies.

Nurses without a recognized certification wishing to use aromatherapy must first complete educational instruction in workshops specifically designed to instruct them in clinically evidence-based aromatherapy application for use on pregnant, laboring and postpartum women. These courses will provide proof of competency and successful completion.

Nurses must maintain and improve their knowledge and competence in relation to aromatherapy as highlighted in specific policies.

The Clinical Manager and Nurse Educator will maintain a list of those staff who are educated in and practicing complementary therapies.

The assessed need, implementation and evaluation of an individual complementary therapy should be documented in the patient's Health Care Record.

The legal and ethical issues of informed consent that clinicians must follow bind all complementary therapies.

The nurse/midwife must accept personal accountability for the practice of aromatherapy.

## Assessment

Information on aromatherapy is to be given to patients in childbirth education and on admission to unit.

Patient education will be provided on clinically evidence-based aromatherapy, and personal aromatherapy will be returned home or locked up with valuables to prevent over- or inappropriate exposure.

The client must be assessed prior to each aromatherapy treatment to ensure no contraindications have developed between treatments. Continual assessment for any changes should made in labor/postpartum.

Aromatherapy treatments are to be documented in patients' notes.

For each patient, an evaluation data sheet needs to be completed using a Likert pre- and post-scale to evaluate treatment response.

The nurse/midwife will only practice aromatherapy treatments subject to the availability of time and the needs of the service. Normal nursing/midwifery commitments must take priority.

**The safety of patients, staff and visitors is our primary concern.**

# Criteria for using aromatherapy in labor
## *Inclusion criteria*

- Women who have been assessed, have no contraindications requiring exclusion and have given verbal consent to treatment.

- Women in pre-established/latent phase or established/active phase of labor.

- Prior to elective or emergency cesarean section.

- Postpartum vaginal or cesarean delivery.

## *Exclusion criteria*

- Preterm labor: lemon spritzer only.

- Women who *do not* give consent.

- Maternal dislike.

- High risk, unstable pregnancy.

- Eclampsia.

- Poor obstetric history.

- Negative medical/obstetric change in condition.

- **Nurses who are pregnant should not perform aromatherapy treatments with oils contraindicated for their stage of pregnancy.**

# Contraindications to aromatherapy use in labor
## *VBAC or previous uterine scar*

- **DO NOT USE** clary sage, rose or jasmine.

## Asthma or hay fever sufferers

- Caution with using lavender or Roman chamomile.

## Diabetes

- **AVOID** eucalyptus.

## Pitocin infusion in progress

- **AVOID** use of clary sage.

## Water birth

- **AVOID** essential oils in the bathtub to prevent contact with and protect baby's eyes. If aromatherapy desired, offer a cotton pad with diluted essential oil for inhalation while in bathtub.

## Allergies to citrus fruits

- **AVOID** use of mandarin, lemon, bergamot.

## Epidural anesthesia

- Use inhalation methods only.
- When aromatherapy oils have been used for back massage, wash and dry back thoroughly prior to epidural insertion.
- **AVOID** clary sage and lavender (sedative/hypotensive oils) after epidural until blood pressure normalizes.

## Resources

Essential oils should always be purchased from a reputable supplier with gas chromatography/mass spectorometry (GCMS) chemical analysis and MSDS information for individual essential oils – see list of companies below.

Essential oils will be ordered by a qualified nurse aromatherapist and will be stored in a locked cabinet with access solely for educated staff.

### *Bottles, inhalers and supplies*

- Arlys: www.arlysnaturals.com

- Massage Warehouse: www.massagewarehouse.com

- SKS Bottle & Packaging, Inc.: www.sks-bottle.com

- Specialty Bottle: www.specialtybottle.com

### *Essential oils in hospital nursing or midwifery clinical aromatherapy programs*

- Absolute Aromas Canada: www.absolute-aromas.ca

- Absolute Aromas UK: www.absolute-aromas.com

- Arlys: www.arlysnaturals.com

- Aromatics International: www.aromatics.com

- Florihana (France): www.florihana.com

- Materia Aromatica: www.materiaaromatica.com

- Nature's Gift: www.naturesgift.com

- NHR Organic Oils (UK): www.nhrorganicoils.com

- Purple Flame (UK): www.purpleflame.co.uk

- Stillpoint Aromatics: www.stillpointaromatics.com

## Nursing, midwifery and aromatherapy organizations

- Alliance of International Aromatherapists: www.alliance-aromatherapists.org

- American Holistic Nurses Association (AHNA): www.ahna.org

- Association of Women's Health, Obstetric and Neonatal Nurses (AWHONN): www.awhonn.org

- Canadian Federation of Aromatherapy (CFA): www.cfacanada.com

- International Confederation of Midwives (ICM): www.internationalmidwives.org

- International Federation of Professional Aromatherapists (IFPA) (UK): www.ifparoma.org

- National Association for Holistic Aromatherapy (NAHA): www.naha.org

- Royal College of Midwives (RCM) (UK): www.rcm.org.uk

## Educational women's health aromatherapy courses for nurses and midwives

- Aromas for Healing: Clinically evidence-based women's health aromatherapy for nurses, midwives, doulas and therapists: www.aromasforhealing.com

- Expectancy: Natural therapies for natural births: www.expectancy.co.uk

- Author's Facebook group: Aromatip of the Month for Health and Happiness: www.facebook.com/groups/165629196795770

# References

Abbaspoor, Z. and Mohammadkhani, S.L. (2013) "Lavender aromatherapy massages in reducing labor pain and duration of labor: A randomized controlled trial." *African Journal of Pharmacy and Pharmacology 7*, 8, 426–430.

Afshar, M.K., Moghadam, Z.B., Taghizadeh, Z., Bekhradi, R., Montazeri, A. and Mokhtari, P. (2015) "Lavender fragrance essential oil and the quality of sleep in postpartum women." *Iranian Red Crescent Medical Journal 17*, 4, e25880.

Agustie, P.R. *et al.* (2017) "Effect of oxytocin massage using lavender essential oil on prolactin level and breast milk production in primiparous mothers after caesarean delivery." *Belitung Nursing Journal 3*, 4, 337–344.

Agustina, C., Hadi, H. and Widyawati, M.N. (2016) "Aromatherapy Massage as an Alternative in Reducing Cortisol Level and enhancing Breastmilk Production on Primiparous Postpartum Women in Semarang." *Asian Academic Society International Conference.*

Apay, S.E., Arslan, S., Akpinar, R.B. and Celebioglu, A. (2012) "Effect of aromatherapy massage on dysmenorrhea in Turkish students." *Pain Management Nursing 13*, 4, 236–240.

Asazawa, A.D., Kato, Y., Yamaguchi, A. and Inoue, A. (2017) "The effect of aromatherapy treatment on fatigue and relaxation for mothers during the early puerperal period in Japan: A pilot study." *International Journal of Community Based Nursing and Midwifery 5*, 4, 365–375.

Bakhtshirin, F., Abedi, S., YusefiZoj, P. and Razmjooee, D. (2015) "The effect of aromatherapy massage with lavender oil on severity of primary dysmenorrhea in Arsanjan students." *Iranian Journal of Nursing and Midwifery Research 20*, 1, 156–160.

Buckle, A. (2001) "The role of aromatherapy in nursing care." *Nursing Clinics of North America 36*, 1, 57–72.

Burns, E., Zobbi, V., Panzeri, D., Oskrochi, R. and Regalia, A. (2007) "Aromatherapy in childbirth: A pilot randomized controlled trial." *BJOG* *114*, 7, 838–844.

Burns, E.E., Blamey, C., Ersser, S.J., Barnetson, L. and Lloyd, A.J. (2000) "An investigation into the use of aromatherapy in intrapartum midwifery practice." *Journal of Alternative and Complementary Medicine 6*, 2, 141–147.

Chen, P.J., Chou, C.C., Yang, L., Tsai, Y.L., Chang, Y.C. and Liaw, J.J. (2017) "Effects of aromatherapy massage on pregnant women"s stress and immune function: A longitudinal, prospective, randomized controlled trial." *Journal of Alternative and Complementary Medicine 23*, 10, 778–786.

Choi, S.Y., Kang, P., Lee, H.S. and Seol, G.H. (2014) "Effects of inhalation of essential oil of Citrus aurantium l var. amara on menopausal symptoms, stress, and estrogen in postmenopausal women: A randomized controlled trial." *Evidence-Based Complementary and Alternative Medicine*, Epub 2014:796518.

Collins Sharp, B.A., Taylor, D.L., Thomas, K.K., Killeen, M.B. and Dawood, M.Y. (2002) "Cyclic perimenstrual pain and discomfort: The scientific basis for practice." *Journal of Obstetric, Gynecological, and Neonatal Nursing 31*, 6, 637–649.

Conrad, P. and Adams, C. (2012) "The effects of clinical aromatherapy for anxiety and depression in the high-risk postpartum woman—A pilot study." *Complementary Therapies in Clinical Practice 18*, 3, 164–168.

Darsareh, F., Taavoni, S., Joolaee, S. and Haghani, H. (2012) "Effect of aromatherapy massage on menopausal symptoms: A randomized placebo-controlled clinical trial." *Menopause 19*, 9, 995–999.

Dhany, A.L., Mitchell, T. and Foy, C. (2012) "Aromatherapy and massage intrapartum service impact on use of analgesia and anesthesia in women in labor: A retrospective case note analysis." *Journal of Alternative and Complementary Medicine 18*, 10, 932–938.

Effati-Daryani, F., Mohammad-Alizadeh-Charandabi, S., Mirgafourvand, M., Taghizadeh, M. and Mohammadi, A. (2015) "Effect of lavender cream with or without foot-bath on anxiety, stress and depression in pregnancy: A randomized placebo-controlled trial." *Journal of Caring Sciences 4*, 1, 63–73.

Eisenberg, D.M., Davis, R.B., Ettner, S.L., Appel, S. *et al.* (1998) "Trends in alternative medicine use in the United States, 1990–1997: Results of a follow-up national survey." *Journal of the American Medical Association 280*, 18, 1569–1576.

Go, G.Y. and Park, H. (2017) "Effects of aroma inhalation therapy on stress, anxiety, depression, and the autonomic nervous system in high-risk pregnant women." *Korean Journal of Women Health Nursing 23*, 1, 33–41.

Grand View Research (2017) *Aromatherapy Market Analysis by Product (Essential Oils, Carrier Oils, Equipment), by Mode of Delivery (Topical, Aerial, Direct Inhalation), by Application, and Segment Forecasts, 2018–2025.* Accessed on November 13, 2018 at https://www.grandviewresearch.com/industry-analysis/aromatherapy-market

Hadi, N. and Hanid, A.A. (2011) "Lavender essence for post-cesarean pain." *Pakistan Journal of Biological Sciences 14*, 11, 664–667.

Halbreich, U. (2003) "The etiology, biology, and evolving pathology of premenstrual syndromes." *Psychoneuroendocrinology 28*, Suppl. 3, 55–99.

Hammad, T.A. (2006) "Suicidality in pediatric patients treated with antidepressant drugs." *Archives of General Psychiatry 63*, 3, 332–339.

Han, S.H., Hur, M.H., Buckle, J., Choi, J. and Lee, M.S. (2006) "Effect of aromatherapy on symptoms of dysmenorrhea in college students: A randomized placebo controlled trial." *Journal of Alternative and Complementary Medicine 12*, 6, 535–541.

Hersh, A.L., Stefanick, M.L. and Stafford, R.S. (2004) "National use of postmenopausal hormone therapy: annual trends and response to recent evidence." *JAMA 291, 1*, 47–53.

Hosseini, S., Heydari, A., Vakili, M., Moghadam, S. and Tazyky, S. (2016) "Effect of lavender essence inhalation on the level of anxiety and blood cortisol in candidates for open-heart surgery." *Iranian Journal of Nursing and Midwifery Research 21*, 4, 397–401.

Hur, M.H., Lee, M.S., Seong, K.Y. and Lee, M.K. (2012) "Aromatherapy massage on the abdomen for alleviating menstrual pain in high school girls: A preliminary controlled clinical study." *Evidence-Based Complementary and Alternative Medicine*, Epub 2012:187163.

Hur, M.H., Yang, Y.S. and Lee, M.S. (2008) "Aromatherapy massage affects menopausal symptoms in Korean climacteric women: A pilot-controlled clinical trial." *Evidence-Based Complementary and Alternative Medicine 5*, 3, 325–328.

Igarashi, T. (2013) "Physical and psychological effects of aromatherapy inhalation on pregnant women: A randomized controlled trial." *Journal of Alternative and Complementary Medicine 19*, 10, 805–810.

Imura, M., Misao, H. and Ushijima, H. (2006) "The psychological effects of aromatherapy-massage in healthy postpartum mothers." *Journal of Midwifery and Women's Health 51*, 2, e21–27.

Johnson, P.J., Kozhimannil, K.B., Jou, J., Ghildayal, N. and Rockwood, T.H. (2016) "Complementary and alternative medicine use among women of reproductive age in the United States." *Women's Health Issues 26*, 1, 40–47.

Ju, H., Jones, M. and Mishra, G. (2014) "The prevalence and risk factors of dysmenorrhea." *Epidemiologic Reviews 36*, 104–113.

Kazemzadeh, R., Nikjou, R., Rostamnegad, M. and Nourouzi, H. (2016) "Effect of lavender aromatherapy on menopause hot flushing: A crossover randomized clinical trial." *Journal of the Chinese Medical Association 79*, 9, 489–492.

Khadivzadeh, T. and Ghabel, M. (2012) "Complementary and alternative medicine use in pregnancy in Mashhad, Iran, 2007–8." *Iranian Journal of Nursing and Midwifery Research 17*, 4, 263–269.

Kheirkhah, M., Vali Pour, N.S., Nisani, L. and Haghani, H. (2014) "Comparing the effects of aromatherapy with rose oils and warm foot bath on anxiety in the first stage of labor in nulliparous women." *Iranian Red Crescent Medical Journal 16*, 9, e14455.

Kianpour, M., Mansouri, A., Mehrabi, T. and Asghari, G. (2016) "Effect of lavender scent inhalation on prevention of stress, anxiety and depression in the postpartum period." *Iranian Journal of Nursing and Midwifery Research 21*, 2, 197–201.

Kim, S., Song, J.A., Kim, M.E. and Hur, M.H. (2016) "Effects of aromatherapy on menopausal symptoms, perceived stress and depression in middle-aged women: A systematic review." *Journal of Korean Academy of Nursing 46*, 5, 619–629.

Lee, K.B., Cho, E. and Kang, Y.S. (2014) "Changes in 5-hydroxytryptamine and cortisol plasma levels in menopausal women after inhalation of clary sage oil." *Phytotherapy Research 28*, 11, 1599–1605.

Lee, M.K. and Hur, M.H. (2011) "Effects of the spouse"s aromatherapy massage on labor pain, anxiety and childbirth satisfaction for laboring women." *Korean Journal of Women Health Nursing 17*, 3, 195–204.

Lee, S.H. (2002) "Effects of aromatherapy massage on depression, self-esteem, climacteric symptoms in the middle aged women." *Korean Journal of Women Health Nursing 8*, 2, 278–288.

Lee, S.O. and Hwang, J.H. (2011) "Effects of aroma inhalation method on subjective quality of sleep, state anxiety, and depression in mothers following cesarean section delivery." *Journal of Korean Academy of Fundamentals of Nursing 18*, 1, 54.

Marzouk, T.M.F., El-Nemer, A.M.R. and Baraka, H.N. (2013) "The effect of aromatherapy abdominal massage on alleviating menstrual pain in nursing students: A prospective randomized cross-over study." *Evidence-Based Complementary and Alternative Medicine*, Epub 2013:742421.

Matsumoto, T., Asakura, H. and Hayashi, T. (2012) "Increased salivary chromogranin A in women with severe negative mood states in the premenstrual phase." *Journal of Psychosomatic Obstetrics and Gynaecology 33*, 3, 120–128.

Matsumoto, T., Asakura, H. and Hayashi, T. (2013) "Does lavender aromatherapy alleviate premenstrual emotional symptoms? A randomized crossover trial." *Biopsychosocial Medicine 7*, 1, 12.

Matsumoto, T., Kimura, T. and Hayashi, T. (2017) "Does Japanese citrus fruit yuzu (Citrus junos Sieb. ex Tanaka) fragrance have lavender-like therapeutic effects that alleviate premenstrual emotional symptoms? A single-blind randomized crossover study." *Journal of Alternative and Complementary Medicine 23*, 6, 461–470.

Metawie, M.A.H., Amasha, H.A., Abdraboo, R.A. and Ali, S.A. (2013) "Effectiveness of aromatherapy with lavender oil in relieving post caesarean incision pain." *Journal of Surgery 3*, 2–1, 8–13.

Mikaningtyas, E. *et al.* (2017) "Lacta Massage using Fennel Essential oil to increase Prolactin Hormone Levels in Postpartum Mothers." *International Journal of Science and Research.*

Milewicz, A. and Jedrzejuk, D. (2006) "Premenstrual syndrome: From etiology to treatment." *Maturitas 55*, Suppl. 1, S47–54.

Murakami, S., Shirota, T., Hayashi, S. and Ishizuka, B. (2005) "Aromatherapy for outpatients with menopausal symptoms in obstetrics and gynecology." *Journal of Alternative and Complementary Medicine 11*, 3, 491–494.

Namazi, M., Amir Ali Akbaria, S., Mojab, F., Talebi, A., Alavi Majd, H. and Jannesari, S. (2014) "Aromatherapy with citrus aurantium oil and anxiety during the first stage of labor." *Iranian Red Crescent Medical Journal 16*, 6, e18371.

Nikjou, R., Kazemzadeh, R., Rostamnegad, M., Moshfegi, S., Karimollahi, M. and Salehi, H. (2016) "The effect of lavender aromatherapy on the pain severity of primary dysmenorrhea: A triple-blind randomized clinical trial." *Annals of Medical and Health Sciences Research 6*, 4, 211–215.

Nobel Prize (2004) "The Nobel Prize in Physiology or Medicine 2004." Accessed on October 15, 2018 at www.nobelprize.org/prizes/medicine/2004/summary

Olapour, A., Behaeen, K., Akhondzadeh, R., Soltani, F., al Sadat Razavi, F. and Bekhradi, R. (2013) "The effect of inhalation of aromatherapy blend containing lavender essential oil on cesarean postoperative pain." *Anesthesiology and Pain Medicine 3*, 1, 203–207.

Ou, M.C., Hsu, T.F., Lai, A.C., Lin, Y.T. and Lin, C.C. (2012) "Pain relief assessment by aromatic essential oil massage on outpatients with primary dysmenorrhea: A randomized, double-blind clinical trial." *Journal of Obstetrics and Gynaecology Research 38*, 5, 817–822.

Pallivalapila, A.R., Stewart, D., Shetty, A., Pande, B., Singh, R. and McLay, J.S. (2015) "Use of complementary and alternative medicines during the third trimester." *Obstetrics and Gynecology 125*, 1, 204–211.

Peng, W., Adams, J., Hickman, L. and Sibbritt, D.W. (2014) "Complementary/ alternative and conventional medicine use amongst menopausal women: Results from the Australian Longitudinal Study on Women"s Health." *Maturitas 79*, 3, 340–342.

Raisi Dehkordi, Z., Hosseini Baharanchi, F.S. and Bekhradi, R. (2014) "Effect of lavender inhalation on the symptoms of primary dysmenorrhea and the amount of menstrual bleeding: A randomized clinical trial." *Complementary Therapies in Medicine 22*, 2, 212–219.

Rapkin, A.J. and Akopians, A.L. (2012) "Pathophysiology of premenstrual syndrome and premenstrual dysphoric disorder." *Menopause International 18*, 2, 52–59.

Rashidi-Fakari, F., Tabatabaeichehr, M., Kamali, H., Rashidi-Fakari, F. and Naseri, M. (2015) "Effect of inhalation of aroma of geranium essence on anxiety and physiological parameters during first stage of labor in nulliparous women: A randomized clinical trial." *Journal of Caring Sciences 4*, 2, 135–141.

Rashidi-Fakari, F., Tabatabaeichehr, M. and Mortazavi, H. (2015) "The effect of aromatherapy by essential oil of orange on anxiety during labor: A randomized clinical trial." *Iranian Journal of Nursing and Midwifery Research 20*, 6, 661–664.

Sadeghi Aval Shahr, H., Saadat, M., Kheirkhah, M. and Saadat, E. (2015) "The effect of self-aromatherapy massage of the abdomen on the primary dysmenorrhea." *Journal of Obstetrics and Gynaecology 35*, 4, 382–385.

Seo, H.K. and Park, K.S. (2003) "A study on the effects of aroma inhalation method using clarysage essential oil on stress in middle-aged women." *Korean Journal of Women Health Nursing 9*, 1, 70–79.

Sharma, P., Malhotra, C., Taneja, D.K. and Saha, R. (2008) "Problems related to menstruation amongst adolescent girls." *Indian Journal of Pediatrics 75*, 2, 125–129.

Shinohara, K., Doi, H., Kumagai, C., Sawano, E. and Tarumi, W. (2017) "Effects of essential oil exposure on salivary estrogen concentration in perimenopausal women." *Neuro Endocrinology Letters 37*, 8, 567–572.

Sibbald, B. (2004) "Rofecoxib (Vioxx) voluntarily withdrawn from market." *Canadian Medical Association Journal 171*, 9, 1027–1028.

Sibbritt, D.W., Catling, C.J., Adams, J., Shaw, A.J. and Homer, C.S. (2014) "The self-prescribed use of aromatherapy oils by pregnant women." *Women and Birth 27*, 1, 41–45.

Son, H.O. and Kim, H.N. (2013) "Effects of aroma back massage on the relief of middle-aged women"s stress." *Journal of the Korean Society of Esthetics and Cosmeceutics 8*, 2, 111–123.

Sut, N. and Kahyaoglu-Sut, H. (2017) "Effect of aromatherapy massage on pain in primary dysmenorrhea: A meta-analysis." *Complementary Therapies in Clinical Practice 27*, 5–10.

Taavoni, S., Darsareh, F., Joolaee, S. and Haghani, H. (2013) "The effect of aromatherapy massage on the psychological symptoms of postmenopausal Iranian women." *Complementary Therapies in Medicine 21*, 3, 158–163.

Tanvisut, R., Kuntharee, T. and Theera, T. (2017) "Efficacy of aromatherapy for reducing pain during labor: A randomized controlled trial." *Archives of Gynecology and Obstetrics 297*, 5, 1145–1150.

Tiran, D. (2016) *Aromatherapy in Midwifery Practice.* London: Singing Dragon.

U.S. Food and Drug Administration (2004) FDA News. "FDA Issues Public Health Advisory on Vioxx as its Manufacturer Voluntarily Withdraws the Product." September 30, 2004. www.fda.gov.

Uysal, M., Doğru, H.Y., Sapmaz, E., Tas, U. *et al.* (2016) "Investigating the effect of rose essential oil in patients with primary dysmenorrhea." *Complementary Therapies in Clinical Practice 24*, 45–49.

Uzuncakmak, T. and Alkaya, S.A. (2017) "Effect of aromatherapy on coping with premenstrual syndrome: A randomized controlled trial." *Complementary Therapies in Medicine 36*, 63–67.

Vakilian, K., Atarha, M., Bekhradi, R. and Charman, R. (2011) "Healing advantages of lavender essential oil during episiotomy recovery: A clinical trial." *Complementary Therapies in Clinical Practice 17*, 1, 50–53.

Vargesson, N. (2015) "Thalidomide-induced teratogenesis: History and mechanisms." *Birth Defects Research, Part C Embryo Today: Reviews 105*, 2, 140–156.

Vaziri, F., Shiravani, M., Najib, F.S., Pourahmad, S., Salehi, A. and Yazdanpanahi, Z. (2017) "Effect of lavender oil aroma in the early hours of postpartum period on maternal pains, fatigue, and mood: A randomized clinical trial." *International Journal of Preventive Medicine 8*, 29.

Watanabe, E., Kuchta, K., Kimura, M., Rauwald, H.W., Kamei, T. and Imanishi, J. (2015) "Effects of bergamot essential oil aromatherapy on mood states, parasympathetic nervous system activity, and salivary cortisol levels in 41 healthy females." *Forschende Komplementarmedizin 22*, 1, 43–49.

Wei, G., Greaver, L.B., Marson, S.M., Herndon, C.H., Rogers, J. and Robeson Healthcare Corporation (2008) "Postpartum depression: Racial differences and ethnic disparities in a tri-racial and bi-ethnic population." *Maternal and Child Health Journal 12*, 6, 699–707.

Wittchen, H.-U., Becker, E., Lieb, R. and Krause, P. (2002) "Prevalence, incidence and stability of premenstrual dysphoric disorder in the community." *Psychological Medicine 32*, 1, 119–132.

Yavari, K.P., Safajou, F., Shahnazi, M. and Nazemiyeh, H. (2014) "The effect of lemon inhalation aromatherapy on nausea and vomiting of pregnancy: A double-blinded, randomized, controlled clinical trial." *Iranian Red Crescent Medical Journal 16*, 3, e14360.

Yazdkhasti, M. and Pirak, A. (2016) "The effect of aromatherapy with lavender essence on severity of labor pain and duration of labor in primiparous women." *Complementary Therapies in Clinical Practice 25*, 81–86.

Yokoyama, K. and Araki, S. (1994) *A Manual of the Japanese Translation of POMS.* Tokyo: Kaneko Shobo.